MICRO MAN
Computers and the Evolution of Consciousness

Dr. Gordon Pask
with Susan Curran

MACMILLAN PUBLISHING CO., INC.

NEW YORK

This book was devised and produced by Multimedia Publications (UK) Ltd.

Editor: Anne Cope
Production: Arnon Orbach
Design and art direction: Millions Design
Illustrations: Millions Design
Picture Research: Andrea Moore, Marion Drescher, Miranda Innes, Brian Reffin-Smith
Indexing: Indexing Specialists

Macmillan Publishing Co., Inc.
866 Third Avenue, New York, N.Y. 10022
Collier Macmillan Canada, Inc.

Library of Congress Cataloging in Publication Data

Pask, Gordon.
Micro man: computers and the evolution of consciousness
Includes index
1. Computers. 2. Brain. 3. Computers and civilization
I. Curran, Susan. II. Title.
QA76.P36   1982   303.4'834   82-9882
ISBN 0-02-595110-6   AACR2

First American Edition 1982
10   9   8   7   6   5   4   3   2   1

Printed by Printer Industria Grafica S.A., Spain.

CONTENTS

INTRODUCTION

This is not a book about computers. It is a book about the developing relationship between human beings and computers. We humans have shaped computers, and now computers are shaping us and our environment.

Computers have evolved remarkably since the invention of the first programmable electronic machines during and immediately after World War II. The invention of the transistor, and the subsequent development of microelectronics, mean that computers and the computing devices we call microprocessors are now small, cheap, reliable and plentiful. The rapid proliferation of computation, communication and control devices is coming to form what we call the 'information environment'. We believe, however, that the change is not merely quantitative. Underlying it are much deeper qualitative changes in the relationship between machines and human beings. These changes, we believe, are leading to the evolution of a new species, a species we have dubbed 'micro man'.

When people build new tools – shovels or bulldozers or computers – they are influenced by the possibilities, often unexpected, opened up by using these tools. Their ideas evolve as result of their interaction with the tool; and as a result, the tool evolves into something which reflects those changing ideas.

Until recently, computers were designed and built by human beings, with the aid of fairly simple tools. Then people began to use more complex machines – like computers themselves – as an aid to this design process. Today computers can design, and microprocessor-controlled machinery can build, computers with little or no human intervention. Computers are no longer merely our tools. They are a species in their own right, neither independent from us, nor subservient to us.

As a result there now exists a medium for computation and information transfer that, like it or not, is evolving by itself. What kind of relationship will exist between the two populations, human and computer? Will it be one of antagonism or co-operation? Our hope – and our belief – is that the two species will co-operate, and that by doing so they will continue to enrich each other's continuing evolution. From this mutual accord there could emerge a metamorphosis, a transformation both of the human mind and of the nature of computing, leading to the genesis of a novel, interdependent pair of species.

We could go even further, and speak not of two species – humans and computers – but of one species, mind, which may reside in one or many people, or machines, or constructs as yet unimagined. We look in this book at some of the similarities, and some of the differences, between what we know of the human brain, and what we know of the 'thought' processes of elaborately programmed computers. It is our belief that just as the boundary between living and non-living things is becoming increasingly blurred, so the distinction between human thought and machine thought is becoming untenable. We envisage a revolutionary expansion of mind, be it individual, social, or wrought in material-other-than-brain-stuff.

Before contemplating expansion, though, we must understand the limitations which govern our present reality. At present, the computer is limited in two ways: by its architecture – the ways in which it can manipulate numbers and symbols – and by the fact that not all of reality can be modelled in terms of numbers and symbols open to logical manipulation. Essentially, current computing operations are founded on the idea of sequence, the notion of attending to one thing after another. This pattern can be seen either as a time sequence, or as a cause-and-effect sequence. In either case, it might be modelled by a piece of string stretched taut, representing the linear nature of causation or time, with knots tied in it to represent the instants of causation or time.

This simple string-and-knot model reflects a long-held view – in the West at least – of the way in which human thought processes work. And indeed in the centuries between the birth of Galileo and Einstein's Theory of Relativity, orderly, sequential and deductive thought scored its greatest triumphs in providing a coherent and logical explanation of the Universe. A little consideration, however, shows up the shortcomings of the string-and-knot model in today's world. It can be useful to talk or write as if we attend to one thing at once. But, in fact, we assume the presence of a 'we' in another dimension, which decides what we attend to, and enables us to switch the focus of our attention. And any form of thought – creative, imaginative, inventive – other than the strictly logical-causative demands the ability to hold several ideas in the mind at once, and to manipulate them in an other-than-sequential way.

We suggest that founding computation on an idealized Western model of sequential, logical, deductive thought has tended to limit the computer's applications. Its manipulations are programmed primarily in a logical way, and it is assumed that the computer cannot possibly create, invent or analogize.

We feel that this restriction is quite unnecessary. There are ways of designing and programming computers or networks of computers which overcome it – we look at some in this book. And we believe these ways will increasingly be adopted in the information environment of the future, enabling the computer to think in ways other than the logical-sequential, and to control environments which cannot be modelled in a serial fashion. It is at this point that a productive interface between computers and the simultaneities and discontinuities of human thought processes becomes possible.

The stage at which computers can think, converse and act like human beings is still a long way off, and there are some who still believe it will never come. We do not underestimate the difficulties, but we believe that artificial intelligence holds limitless possibilities, and that machine brains, alone or in populations, may come to surpass the abilities of the human brain in more and more fields. The implications of this are both exciting and frightening. We acknowledge the dangers. But with wisdom, a certain sense of adventure, and maybe a certain courage, we shall see a world far richer in human possibility, still with a human tradition, and beautiful beyond imagination.

This is the world of micro man. It is taking shape today, and increasingly, in a variety of disciplines from psychology to architecture, from education to epistemology, we can trace the emergence of men and women whose ideas exemplify this new era. One aim of this book is to bring together their theses, at least in outline, and to indicate how a coherent set of ideas, shaping and shaped by the development of computing, underlies them. Another aim is to help you, the reader, to become familiar with this new world. For it is your world that is being shaped, and you who must play a part in shaping it.

Chapter **1 COMPUTERS COME OF AGE**

To vast numbers of computer programmers and operators the computer is a large, powerful, and sometimes exasperating calculating machine. But it is actually and potentially much more than that.

A modern computer is very simple and very complicated, simple because all it really does is add, subtract and compare, and complicated because all the tasks required of it must be reducible to these simple operations.

Computing began with counting, and counting began with the realization that 'one' is different from 'two' or 'many' and that there is an important similarity between, say, 'two cows' and 'two sheep' and an important difference between 'two cows' and 'three cows'. Once quantity is divorced from quality it becomes possible to play with symbols of quantity (numbers) and thereby to calculate. Numbers can be manipulated in ways that objects cannot. What is the square root of a cow? The question is meaningless, but the square root of a number is meaningful in our system of mathematics.

In the great space of time between the invention of the abacus and the invention of punched card machinery in the nineteenth century human ingenuity was devoted to automating calculation, to making the manipulation of numbers more accurate and less tedious. In fact the path of computation did not diverge from that of calculation until the mid-nineteenth century. A computer, as distinct from a calculator, can manipulate many kinds of symbols including numbers, provided they are used according to an agreed system, and it does so in an infinitely variable number of ways. In the sense that we humans are superb manipulators of symbols, we too are computers.

What, fundamentally, is the purpose of manipulating signs and symbols? To communicate, or control, or both. The developing relationship between computation, communication and control more than anything explains how the computer has developed and where it is likely to lead us in the future. Computing, because it obliges us to re-examine our notions of communication, control, memory, distance and time, is transforming our late twentieth century world just as surely as the discovery of number transformed the world of our remote ancestors.

The mechanization of arithmetic

Charting the motions of the planets. Of all the sciences, astronomy requires the most exact and the most repetitive calculations. Would a pocket calculator have accelerated the discoveries of a Copernicus or a Kepler or a Newton?

Let us contrast for a moment a modern electronic computer and a simple calculating device like the abacus. The computer user does not actively supervise each individual step of the computer's operations; control is delegated to a program, to a set of instructions carried out automatically. And even to the machine's designers it may not be clear exactly what the machine is doing at a given moment. The modern computer is a 'black box'. The abacus user by contrast slides beads along wires at each stage of calculation and can see exactly what is going on. The history of computing is one of increasing delegation of control and increasing machine inscrutability. Every increase in automation has required a corresponding increase in man-machine communication. We have had to find ways of telling machines what to do, and when they have

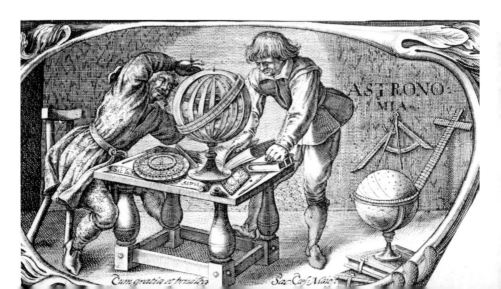

completed their obscure ballet, they have to tell us the result. They must interface with us at a practical level (we put something in, take something out) and at an intelligible level (they must make sense of what we put in, and we must understand what they put out).

Put at its simplest, a modern computer manipulates symbols by adding, subtracting and comparing them, and it does so via instructions known as a program. The entire complex world of mathematical manipulation can be broken down into adding and subtracting (actually these can be simplified still further into just one operation, but that is another story). Multiplication becomes a matter of repeatedly adding, and division of repeatedly subtracting. More complex calculations can be handled by a variety of techniques. Logarithms, for example, help to break operations down into addition and subtraction. Comparison is of vital importance if the computer is to follow instructions; it must be able to check whether two symbols or sequences of symbols are the same or different, since that may determine the instructions that are followed next.

Let us travel quickly along stretches of the road that led to the electronic computer. An abacus is not a childish toy. It was invented in China in the thirteenth century and is still used in banks in the Far East today. It was used in Europe, but not to the extent of discouraging mathematicians like Blaise Pascal and Gottfried Wilhelm Leibnitz from inventing complex sets of cogwheels and shafts to mechanize simple calculations. When used by a skilled operator the abacus is very efficient. Tests comparing it with an electrical desk calculator over a range of arithmetical operations have shown it to be just as fast and just as accurate; it can cope with multiplication and division by repeated addition and subtraction.

There are many different designs of abacus but they all work on the same principle. The drawings on page 8 show the modern Japanese form of abacus, the *soroban*, being used to add 862 to 164298. Eight separate actions are needed to do this. On Pascal's calculating machine, invented in 1642, the same sum takes three steps: enter the first number, enter the second, activate the add mechanism. The 'carrying' operation, done by hand on the abacus, was automated. The numbers were entered by moving the wheels with a stylus, and the result was displayed on result wheels. Only two numbers could be manipulated at a time, though, and the result was not always correct. A later calculating machine invented by Leibnitz mechanized multiplication and division as well.

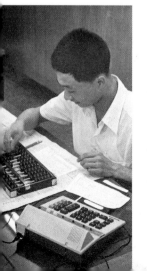

Counter clerk in a Japanese bank – equally adept with the abacus and the electronic calculator.

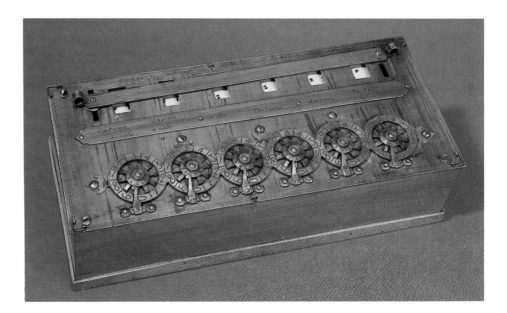

A replica of Pascal's calculating machine. The result cylinders can be seen in the windows above the calculating wheels.

Heaven

Earth

On the Japanese soroban, beads above the beam count as 5 and beads below as 1. Different numbers are produced by moving 'heaven' and 'earth' beads towards the beam. So, in this drawing, the abacus reads 164298. The maximum number that can be represented is 999999999.

0 0 0 1 6 4 2 9 8

The Difference Engine

Some 150 years later Charles Babbage, a British mathematician with a home and workshop in London, designed a machine more important in theory than in practice: the Difference Engine. Its purpose was to calculate tables of mathematical functions, including logarithms, with greater accuracy than had been possible previously.

Babbage's device owed much to earlier calculating machine design, but one of his unique additions was the concept of registers, different locations in the machine in which numbers could be entered and stored. The storage of input was something new. Pascal's machine had only one set of 'setting' wheels and could only hold two numbers at a time. All the input to Babbage's machine – the numbers required for a calculation possibly involving many successive arithmetical operations – was entered into the registers first; the manipulation came later. Babbage's concept of output was also more sophisticated; his machine was going to engrave results on a copper plate that could be printed from directly. At one stroke he provided the user with a record of each result, and circumvented the errors which inevitably occur in setting matter for print.

These four drawings show the steps involved in adding 8623 to 164298.

Drawing 1: to add 2 to 8, clear column 1 (units) and reinstate one bead, then add 1 to column 2 (tens), which makes it up to 10, so clear it and add 1 to column 3 (hundreds).

Drawing 2: to add 20, add 2 to column 2.

Drawing 3: to add 600, add 6 to column 3.

Drawing 4: to add 8000, add 8 to column 4, reinstate two beads, then add 1 to column 5.

Read off the answer: 172921.

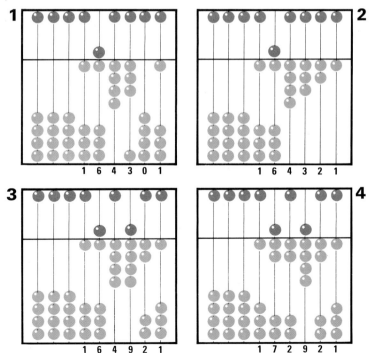

Babbage's Difference Engine. Part of the original uncompleted mechanism of this can be seen in the Science Museum in London, as can part of the original, and also unfinished, Analytical Engine.

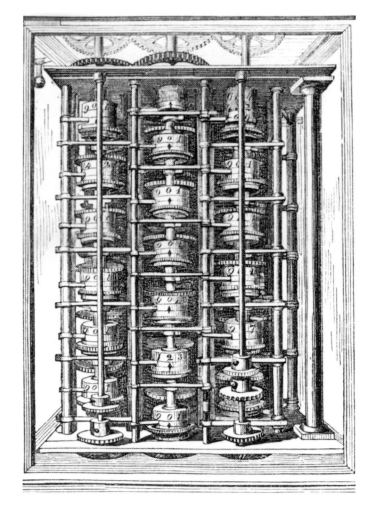

Sadly Babbage's mental ingenuity was not matched by the mechanical expertise of his time. Although he worked on the Difference Engine for a good 20 years, devoting most of his energy to trying to solve the practical problems it generated, he was unable to find an engineer capable of constructing it. Nevertheless the Difference Engine concept had its descendants. A Swedish father and son, Per Georg and Edvard Scheuz, developed a less elaborate device than Babbage's, and even in this century a few mechanical difference engines have found their way into commercial use.

The Analytical Engine

In 1832, still struggling with the technical problems of his Difference Engine, Babbage transferred his attention to a still more ambitious project, the Analytical Engine. Where the Difference Engine was designed to produce mathematical tables and nothing else, the Analytical Engine was designed to carry out virtually any type of calculation. It was designed to store data so that they could be used in any sequence (the Difference Engine's data store could only be used in a fixed sequence); it was also designed to store numbers generated in the course of calculations; and it was designed to be able to accept all sorts of different instructions (the Difference Engine had fixed instructions built into it). In modern terms the Analytical Engine had a read-write memory – data could be read from store and entered into it. It was also programmable – it could be fed with variable instructions as to how data were to be manipulated.

The design of the Analytical Engine made provision for two distinct sub-devices: an arithmetic/logic unit (the 'mill' as Babbage called it) and a control unit. The former manipulated the data according to arithmetical or logical rules, and the latter interpreted the instructions in the correct sequence and activated the arithmetic/logic unit.

Even in the early nineteenth century, then, the lineaments of the modern computer were emerging. The Analytical Engine and its modern descendants share the following features:

a method of inputting data and instructions;

a memory, for storing information;

a control unit, for carrying out instructions in the right order;

an arithmetic/logic unit, for carrying out the necessary manipulations;

a method of outputting results.

From an engineering point of view, the Analytical Engine was an even more fearsome undertaking than the Difference Engine. Even a simple version of it would have contained over 50 000 moving parts. Babbage insisted on storing 1 000 numbers to no less than 50 decimal places, a ridiculous degree of accuracy. Lord Moulton, a lawyer and mathematician, drew a touching picture of the man who had too many new ideas and ambitions too large for the technology of his time. 'One of the sad memories of my life is a visit to the celebrated mathematician and inventor, Mr. Babbage. He was far advanced in age, but his mind was still as vigorous as ever. He took me through his workrooms. In the first room I saw the parts of the original Calculating Machine, which had been shown in an incomplete state many years before and had even been put to some use. I asked him about its present form. "I have not finished it because in working at it I came on the idea of my Analytical Machine, which would do all that it was capable of doing and much more. Indeed, the idea was so much simpler that it would have taken more work to complete the calculating machine than to design and construct the other in its entirety, so I turned my attention to the Analytical Machine." I asked if I could see it. "I have never completed it" he said, "because I hit upon the idea of doing the same thing by a different and far more effective method, and this rendered it useless to proceed on the old lines." Then we went into the third room. There lay scattered bits of mechanism but I saw no trace of any working machine. Very cautiously I approached the subject and received the dreaded answer, "It is not constructed yet, but I am working at it, and will take less time to construct it altogether than it would have taken to complete the Analytical Machine from the stage in which I left it." I took leave of the old man with a heavy heart.'

Unfortunately Babbage left no clear description of his Analytical Engine and its special features. However a number of his followers, including Lord Byron's daughter, Lady Lovelace, repaired this omission.

Telling the computer what to do

Babbage used punched cards, derived from Jacquard loom cards, for the storage of instructions. The cards, one per instruction, were to be fed into the Analytical Engine in correct sequence, each card triggering off the next instruction in the sequence. There were also separate cards that specified which locations in the data store held the data to be manipulated. The whole pack of cards could be used and re-used, would not take up space in the data store, and could be swapped for a different pack when a different computation was required. Punched cards were enthusiastically adapted to many other types of machine throughout the nineteenth century, including fairground machinery and the pianola, and even today punch card and punch tape machinery is quite widely used.

Thanks to Lady Lovelace we know something of the sophistication that Babbage intended to build into his punched card system. In the Jacquard loom or the pianola roll the ordering of instructions is a simple matter; they are carried out one by one, in the order in which they are fed into the machine. The special problems posed by mathematics, however, made it desirable for more complex ordering to be possible.

Lady Lovelace, writing in 1842, outlined two of the basic

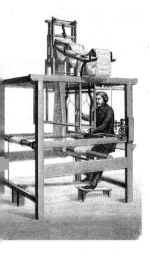

The Jacquard loom, invented by Joseph-Marie Jacquard in France in 1862. The continuous loop of punched cards at the top of the loom controlled the loom mechanism, producing repeat patterns (engraving published in Le Journal de la Jeunesse, Paris, 1876).

features of modern computer programming: the loop and the branch. The idea of the loop is that instructions need only be fed into the machine once. Many mathematical calculations are extremely repetitive in nature. It is therefore necessary to feed the same instructions into the machine over and over again, or to find some way of providing it with long sequences of repeating instructions. A loop of instructions does the latter. A trigger mechanism identifies the last instruction in the sequence and takes the program back to the first instruction automatically.

The idea of a branch is that the result of a particular manipulation may affect the order in which the rest of the instructions are carried out. Let us imagine that a program is looking for a number that fits a certain criterion, the lowest whole number exactly divisible by 4, 7 and 13, say. Diagrammatically the instructions could be set up as shown below. Instructions 2, 3, 4 and 5 form a loop; they are repeated again and again until the answer to the question which forms instruction 3 is 'yes'. Instruction 3 makes a branch in the program: if the answer is 'yes', instruction 6 will follow; if 'no' instruction 4 will follow. With loops and branches the need for human intervention at critical moments is done away with.

Is a program part of the computer or part of the operator? Today computer users tend to act as if the program were part of the computer, not least because virtually all modern computers have some sets of instructions (including language compilers) built into them. To differentiate between machinery and instructions, the former is known as hardware and the latter as software.

The program – the software – causes the computer to carry out the programmer's instructions in a set sequence. The writer of the program may not be aware in what order the machine will actually implement his or her instructions; in fact it is not

A flow chart describing how to find the lowest whole number exactly divisible by 4, 7 and 13. Instructions 2, 3, 4 and 5 form a loop.

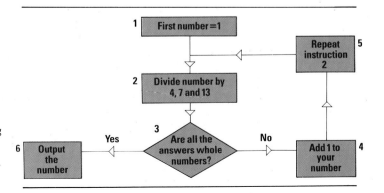

uncommon, in more complex programs, for the programmer to accidentally structure the program in such a way that the computer will never, whatever the data, carry out some of the instructions he or she has written. Nevertheless the computer can only act according to the rules spelled out by the programmer, whether or not the programmer can predict how the program will run. Barring mechanical accident, the computer will execute the same program on the same data in exactly the same way every time.

The facility for the program instructions to be executed in different orders, depending upon the results produced by carrying out earlier instructions in the sequence, is one of the essential features of the modern computer. It is perhaps this, more than anything, which differentiates the computer from the calculator. Programmable calculators can be instructed to carry out sequences of operations; but once the order of the instructions in the sequence becomes variable, they are more properly described as computers.

Algorithms and programming languages

Computer programming techniques have progressed immensely since Babbage's day. Two major advances have been the theory of algorithms, mainly elaborated in the 1950s by the Russian mathematician A. A. Markov, and the concept of program languages.

An algorithm is a set of procedural steps that outlines how a problem is to be solved. For the purposes of computing, an algorithm is a skeleton that is used to construct a program that tells the computer what to do. The simple flow chart on page 13 is itself an algorithm.

A program language is, essentially, a set of conventions that enable human instructions to be converted into codes manipulable by the computer. Ever since Babbage's day calculating machines and computers have worked with information coded into simple two-state or binary codes. Punched cards are an example of binary code: the information they contain exists as holes or the absence of holes in certain patterns. In a modern electronic computer information is represented by pulses of electricity, or the absence of pulses of electricity. In calculators of the immediate pre-electronic era information was held by electromagnetic relays, also capable of existing in only two states. Outside the computer we use 0 and 1 to represent these two states. Numbers, letters and other symbols, whether they represent data or instructions, have to be translated into binary code – there are internationally agreed conventions for doing this – before the computer can manipulate them. Numbers 1 to 10, for example, become 001, 010, 011, 100, 101, 110, 111, 1000, 1001, and 1010 in binary.

Obviously long sequences of instructions translated into ones and zeros become enormously cumbersome – it is extremely difficult and tedious to write programs consisting of interminable strings of ones and zeros. Programming languages get round the problem by replacing binary codes with more manageable and intelligible symbols. Let us suppose that the computer interprets 00010110 as the instruction ADD. At one time the poor programmer would have had to translate such instructions into the appropriate binary codes, but today the job of compiling or interpreting – both ways of translating program languages into binary code – is done by the computer itself, either before the program is run or while it is being run.

Today programming languages are very efficient and powerful and have advanced far beyond the simple add, and subtract and compare instructions into which all computer manipulations can be broken down. They combine whole sequences of arithmetic/logic operations into single higher-level instructions that usually take the form of recognizable words or near-words. These higher-level instructions still have to be translated into binary of course.

From calculation to computing

Babbage was the first man to realize that punched cards could be used to instruct a machine to do calculations. The cards were originally invented to control machinery, specifically the movement of threads in a loom. Later, as we have said, they found all sorts of mechanical applications. And towards the end of the nineteenth century they began to be used not only in calculating machines but also for manipulating non-numerical forms of data.

Comparison is the essential form of manipulation of non-mathematical data. One of the first people to use punched cards for this purpose was Herman Hollerith, a statistician working for the Bureau of the Census in the United States. His idea was to code census information onto punched cards so that it could be analyzed in a fraction of the time it would take human sorters to do the job. The patterns of holes were to be sensed electrically – the presence of a hole allowed current to flow, the absence of a hole stopped it. Hollerith's system was put to the test in the census year of 1890, and was so successful that a sizeable industry of office data processing machinery followed. Punched card machinery is not suitable for elaborate calculations, but it is well suited to the repetitive sorting and arithmetical operations that make up much clerical work in commerce and industry, and

A commemoration of the American census of 1890, the first application of punched card technology to the sorting of statistics.

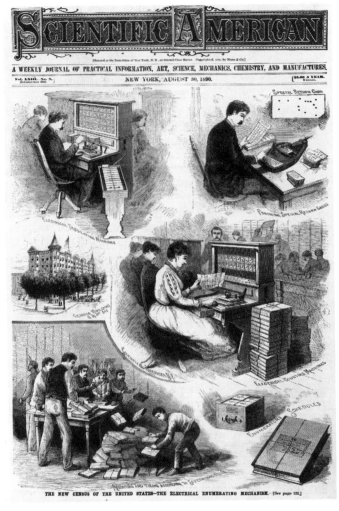

THE NEW CENSUS OF THE UNITED STATES—THE ELECTRICAL ENUMERATING MECHANISM.—[See page 132.]

some in science and technology.

As the punched card office machinery industry grew many of the practical problems that had dogged Babbage were solved. Finally, in the 1940s, two machines were constructed which substantially fulfilled Babbage's dream. One was American, the Automatic Sequence Controlled Calculator, or ASCC, designed by Howard H. Aiken of Harvard University, and built by IBM in 1944. The other was German, a machine designed along similar principles by Konrad Zuse, the Z3, completed in 1941. These were both electromechanical machines, based upon electromagnetic relays. Ironically their day – so long awaited – was to be a short one. In 1945 a new technique, based not on electro-magnetism but on electronics, took over, pioneered by the Electronic Number Integrator and Calculator, E N I A C. This was an American machine and is generally regarded as the first electronic digital computer.

Digital and analog

All the devices we have described so far, from the abacus to ENIAC, have been 'digital'. If you think of the Latin root of the word digital, *digitus* meaning 'finger', and of counting on your fingers you will appreciate that calculation is possible in whole fingers only! Digital machines can only work with discrete numbers. Even if numbers are calculated to many decimal places of accuracy there is still a definite and unmistak-able distance between, say, 1.999 and 2.000. Digital devices work by manipulating these small but identifiable intervals.

An analog device, however, works by representing *directly* the quantities that are being manipulated. A slide rule is an analog device. Calculations made on it are accurate but one cannot say precisely what the answer is, only that it lies somewhere between 1.999 and 2.000. It does not calculate on the basis of clearly defined intervals.

Many real life measurable quantities are analog in nature: time, temperature, pressure and speed, for instance. This is why analog methods are often preferred when these quantities have to be represented in a calculation. Digital quantities were once manipulated by moving sets of gears with teeth which interlock at fixed intervals – the machines of Pascal and Leibnitz worked in this way. The equivalent method of manipulating analog quantities was a gearing device with continually varying ratios. One of the earliest analog calculating machines to use this principle was designed by James Thomson in 1876. A large number of non-mainstream computers (some of which we look at in Chapter 8) have used analog methods. Today, of course, the usual method of representing a continuously variable quantity is not through mechanical gears but by a variable electrical current.

Today's digital computers can cope with analog informa-tion, but they have to convert it into digital form. They do this by measuring the value of the analog quality – say, temperature – at regular intervals and converting that measurement into a number of electrical pulses corresponding to that measurement. In an analog watch, for example, time and the hands on the watch face change continuously; a digital watch, however, converts the passage of time into tiny intervals, marked by the numbers changing on the dial.

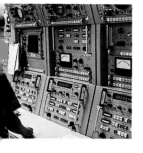

High speed digital recorders linked to a 210 ft (70 m) radio antenna.

Electronic computers

The great stumbling block in refining the mechanical computer was the enormous number of moving parts it required. As often happens, it was the pressure of wartime needs that produced a new solution to the problem – the electronic computer. In the early models, data and instructions were processed not by mechanical movement but by varying electrical signals. The electrical signals were amplified in power and magnitude by thermionic valves (vacuum tubes). Valves could be used (as they were in the radio sets of that period) to convert a small electrical signal into a larger one. Alternatively they could be used as switches triggered by a very small signal to produce a much larger one. In this mode they acted in much the same way as mechanical calculators when triggered by holes in a punched card.

The first two valve computers were Colossus I, designed in the United Kingdom by Alan Turing, Tommy Flowers and Max Newman in 1943, and ENIAC, designed by J.P. Eckert and J.W. Maunchly of the University of Pennsylvania in 1945. Colossus I, and its successor Colossus II, were designed to break enemy codes produced by the German Enigma cryptographic machine. The purpose of Colossus was to compare large numbers of intercepted enemy coded messages in order to discover recurring clusters of letters. These clusters were then analyzed by the human codebreakers of the special Government cypher school at Bletchley Park, Bedfordshire, England. They knew that certain letters in German occurred more than others and, by comparing these with the recurring clusters identified by Colossus, eventually broke the enemy codes.

ENIAC was designed to calculate trajectories of bombs and shells – a process involving complicated interactions between variables such as velocity, mass, air resistance, and the force of gravity. After the war it was adapted to perform many other functions, thus becoming the first general-purpose computer.

The advantage of these early electronic computers was that they could operate much more quickly than their electromagnetic rivals. ENIAC, for example, could do more in an hour than the electromagnetic ASCC could do in a week. But these early electronic machines were bulky, power-hungry and unreliable. ENIAC, for example, covered 3 000 cubic feet (85 cubic metres) and weighed 30 tons (tonnes). It contained 18 000 valves and was difficult to keep going for more than a few minutes at a time. By modern standards its capacity too was severely limited. Its memory capacity was just 20 'words' of 10 figures each, and it could handle only 300 'words' of program instructions.

So expensive were these machines that their makers envisaged a future in which, at best, only a few dozen of them would ever be made. The fact that they were wrong was due to the development of the transistor, a miniature component that performed the same function as the thermionic valve. But before we leave the first electronic computers it is important to remember that, however clumsy they may seem now, they computed on exactly the same principles as those of today.

Turing's machine

It was Alan Turing, the brilliant mathematician and pioneer computer scientist, who first laid down the fundamental principles of computation. In 1937 he described a hypothetical machine composed of an 'automaton' that performed the actual calculations, and a form of data storage, the tape. Data could be stored on the tape, but only in the form of zeros, ones and punctuation symbols. The automaton could read symbols from, or write or delete symbols from, the portion of the tape beneath its read-and-write head. It could also move the tape one step to the left or right.

By a complex mathematical proof, Turing was able to show that, using only three computable functions – addition, subtraction and comparison – his machine could theoretically handle many algebraic and mathematical operations. Provided that the tape was correctly coded, the machine would always come up

ENIAC, a giant infant – hungry, unpredictable, always greedy for attention.

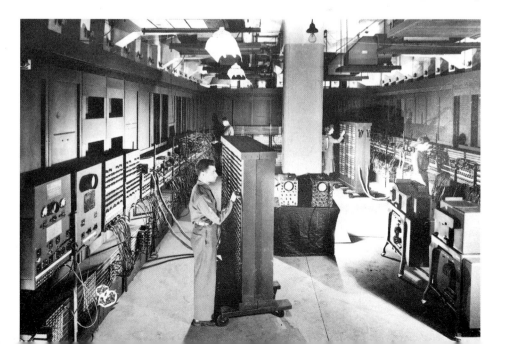

with the correct result. Moreover, it would continue to do so as long as the tape required it to, a fact which gave it a theoretically infinite capacity. These simple principles, carried over into more complicated and efficient types of computer architecture, still govern our present ideas about the fundamental limits of computation.

Modern computers

In many ways, ENIAC and Colossus were the first machines to qualify as computers in the sense that we use the word today. The gulf that separates them from today's machines, however, is not simply technical but one of social and psychological awareness. ENIAC meant nothing to the man in the street; for society at large the impact of its work was minimal. Today, everyone is aware of computers, and virtually everyone comes into contact with their output.

Of course, there are many more computers around today. If no technical developments had taken place since ENIAC and other computers of its generation there would probably be a fair number of these in use today. Their size, cost and unreliability however, would certainly have prevented their use on the same scale as today's computers.

Fortunately, one major invention, and the successive developments that refined and extended it, helped to change the picture. In 1947 a team including John Bardeen, Walter Brattain and William Shockley at Bell Laboratories in New Jersey created the first transistor.

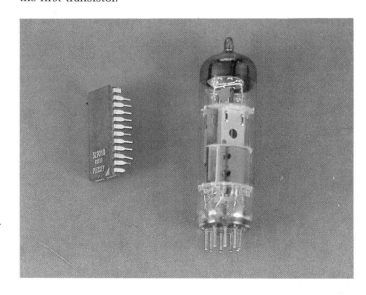

Two generations of electronic technology. Right: the thermionic valve, about 2 in (5 cm) long. Left: a fully packaged memory chip. The chip itself is hermetically sealed inside a plastic case. The metal 'legs' are its electrical connections.

A transistor resembles a sandwich but contains materials which have the property of conducting electricity only at a particular voltage. Because of this, they are often called semiconductors. For appropriate electrical signals, the transistor does the same job as a thermionic valve. It can amplify signals, and also invert their sign, making positive negative or negative positive. Transistors are used as amplifiers in hi-fi equipment and up-to-date analog computers. But they can also be operated in a different and digital mode; as switches or relays with only the stable conditions 'on' or 'off'. In this mode they work as devices that produce an electrical on or off signal. It is also quite a simple matter for transistors to act as latches, to remain on once triggered until a later signal triggers them off.

The transistor has three great advantages over the valve. One, it is small; even the earliest transistors were barely larger than a match head. Two, it is cheap. The first transistorized computers were admittedly no cheaper than their valve-based predecessors, but with modern mass production procedures, the price of a single transistor has become minuscule. And three, it is much more reliable. With these points in its favour, it was inevitable that the transistor would take over from the valve. In 1956 the first fully transistorized computer, the Leprechaun, was built by Bell Laboratories.

Since then transistor development has followed two main lines. First, transistors have become even smaller, a feature that not only enables lots of them to be packed into a small space, but also enhances their speed of operation. Second, there have been steady improvements in linking transistors together.

Initially transistors were linked, as valves had been, by a tangle of wires. The first improvement was to mount the components of the circuit onto a board, and to deposit or etch the wiring onto the board itself. Later, came the fully integrated circuit, in which sets of components and their linkages came to be manufactured in one operation. And in the latest stage, the number of components that can be manufactured in one piece has been massively increased. This very large scale integration, or VLSI, means that thousands of transistors can be packed onto a chip of silicon less than $\frac{1}{4}$ inch (1 cm) square. Today, chips containing 250 000 or more transistors are in mass production.

At the same time, the cost of each component has fallen dramatically. For a few cents it is possible to buy a silicon chip containing circuits offering as much potential computing power as ENIAC. Of course, a silicon chip is not only cheaper but also far more reliable; and being so very much smaller than ENIAC, it costs only a tiny fraction as much to run.

A designer producing the master pattern for all the circuitry required on a single chip. The design is then photographically reduced to chip size ready for etching by laser onto a wafer of silicon.

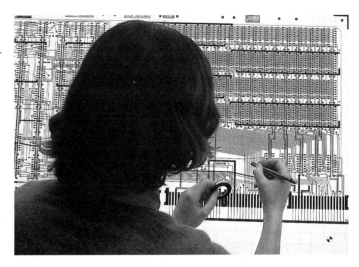

With each plunge in the cost of computers, it became possible to use them for a wider range of applications. In the early days, and even through the 1960s, computing power was so expensive that every computer was used intensively, day and night, for high value-added computing operations. Today, processors are dedicated to the most trivial tasks. At the heart of a quartz wristwatch, for instance, is a silicon chip whose sole job is to count the oscillations of a quartz crystal, and convert the regular time interval between them into seconds, minutes and hours. Processors are routinely used to monitor the temperature in domestic washing machines and central heating controllers. By a simple process of comparison, they test the temperature at regular intervals and compare it to the desired temperature.

These processors are dedicated, programmed to carry out a limited range of specific tasks. The same liberality of use is seen in general-purpose computers. Most people who buy home computers or mini computers do not use them intensively. Despite their sophistication they are so cheap that their owners can use them purely as hobby machines, an attitude unthinkable 20 years ago.

Silicon chips, microprocessors and computers

Miniaturized components which make up circuits able to compute, like those on a silicon chip, are now so common that people talk as though their watch, washing machine or telephone actually contained a computer. In one sense they are right. It may be more appropriate, though, to use the word computer to indicate a general-purpose computing

A Chinese version of the abacus (inset), operated by hand, with every calculation step plainly visible; and the microscopic mystery of hundreds of chips on a wafer-thin disc of silicon. The density of chips that can be packed onto a given area of silicon has roughly doubled every year since 1960.

machine that can be programmed by the user and that has input and output, memory and manipulative ability. In this definition we should include the idea of a separately identifiable machine. There are a number of words we can use for the watch component; perhaps the most precise and useful is 'microprocessor', the term for a chip containing circuits that perform manipulative and control operations inside a computer. However, the microprocessor within the computer will be programmable, while the watch component will not be. Instead its program is contained within its fixed wiring pattern; it is dedicated to a single task, or small range of tasks, and like the Difference Engine it acts as a special-purpose device that operates without the need for program input.

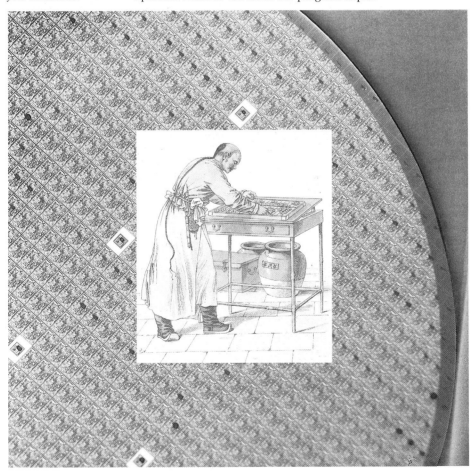

The fine wires that attach a microchip to its soldered electrical connections are made of gold. Magnification here is approximately 500.

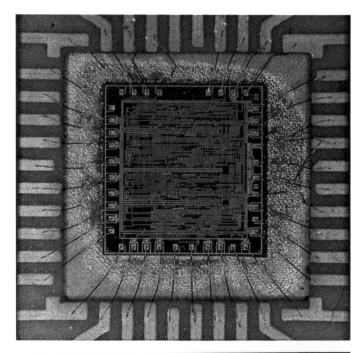

Look inside any small or medium size computer today and you will see a number of chips, in their plastic casings, fixed to a printed circuit board and connected by lots of geometrically laid out wires.

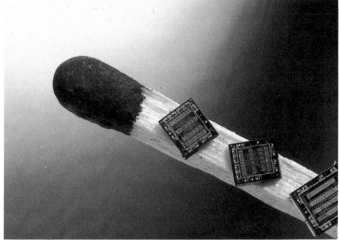

New technologies

Because of the success of the microprocessor, it has become conventional to see computing generally in terms of micro-miniaturized electronic circuits. This has had the effect of stifling computer designs that do not necessarily require electronic components at all. Biotechnology offers one such design possibility. New techniques of handling living cells promise the development of biological media that might act as computing devices. The structure of a cell, for example, might be transformed to process information in a way analogous to a silicon chip. Alternatively, living cells could form the basis of an entirely different machine that might have nothing more in common with more conventional computers than the fact that it computes. We look at some of these more esoteric options in Chapter 8.

Silicon itself is facing competition from alternative mineral compounds, including gallium arsenide. The advantages of such rival materials lie in both manufacture and performance.

A typical small computer system

We shall briefly describe a fairly typical small computer system, and the components that might be associated with it. However, it is essential to remember that none of the devices we describe will necessarily be found in every other computer existing today. Computers may all have the same functions, and the same five functional elements (input, storage, control, arithmetic/logic and output). But they do not necessarily use the same hardware to carry out those functions. And they do not necessarily have the same programs either.

The photograph below shows a typical small computer system: the Apple II. It has sold widely for use in small

The Apple II desk top computer, with keyboard, video monitor and, in this picture, two disc drive units which take small floppy discs. Apple III, its more sophisticated successor, can be connected to larger computers and to other Apples. Apple software packages enable business users to handle word processing, financial planning, sorting and editing of mailing lists, ledger systems, stock control and so on.

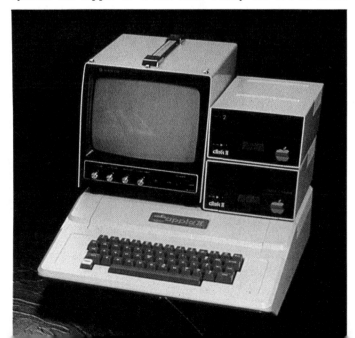

businesses, schools, and at home, and is typical of the sort of personal computer that is well adapted to a general, non-specialist market. What does it consist of?

An input device In this case, data and instructions can be input to the computer via a keyboard. (They can also be 'read' into the computer from its memory devices, but we shall come to that shortly.) The operator simply types on the keyboard (which is similar to a typewriter keyboard, but with a few extra keys) and the information is coded into the on/off binary code the computer uses by a processor linked to the keyboard.

Some ways of storing information Some of the silicon chips inside the computer contain circuits that are designated as 'memory': that is, they act as repositories for data or instructions which are not immediately required for processing. These form an *internal memory* for the computer. The internal memory of a computer like the Apple is both limited and temporary. It is limited by the amount of information it can absorb – between 22 000 and 56 000 words of instruction. It is important to remember that these special computer words are not the same as words in the general linguistic sense. The data stored in some types of internal memory last only so long as the computer is switched on. For this reason it is essential for the computer to be able to draw on greater amounts of permanently stored information. Such information would include particular programs, together with the data needed to run them.

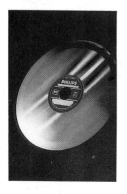

A floppy disc. Even the smallest 'floppies' store between 80 000 and 500 000 characters. Any piece of data can be retrieved in about a fifth of a second, compared with the 10 or 15 minutes it takes to reel through a cassette tape.

Many small computers use standard audio cassette tapes as their storage medium. The data are recorded in sound form onto the tape. They can then be played back at will into the computer, which 'reads' the sound signals. The trouble with tapes, though, is that you have to run right through the tape in order to reach the material at the end of a particular track. A better (and more expensive) storage medium is the floppy disc.

The floppy disc is like a music record. Data are stored in magnetic form along circular tracks on each side of the disc. Data are transmitted to the computer by a reading head in the disc drive. The discs used by this particular computer can each hold 116 000 words of data. Putting a new disc in the drive unit is just like changing a record on a turntable.

Both cassette tapes and floppy discs are read-write forms of memory. The computer can read information off them, enter information onto them, or 'write over' redundant information. Part of the computer's internal memory, on the other hand, is in read-only form. This contains unchanging operating instructions, instructions for decoding languages the computer can understand, and so on, in a form that ensures that the information will not be lost when the computer is switched off. In this model, 6 000 or 8 000 words, approximately, of space is taken up by read-only memory.

A control device and an arithmetic/logic unit The microprocessor chip inside this computer, a model 6502, is shown on page 28 as part of a more sophisticated chip, a model 6500.

An output device The video display unit you can see in the photograph acts as a primary output device, as well as echoing the user's input to the computer. It offers colour graphics, as well as character output. In addition, this computer can be linked to a printer, to provide hard copy output when required.

A one-man stand against the paperless office?

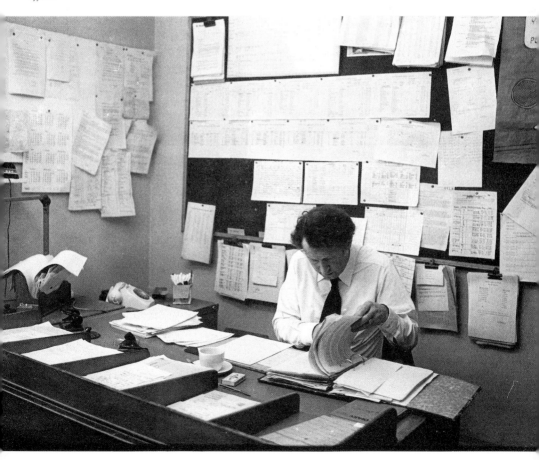

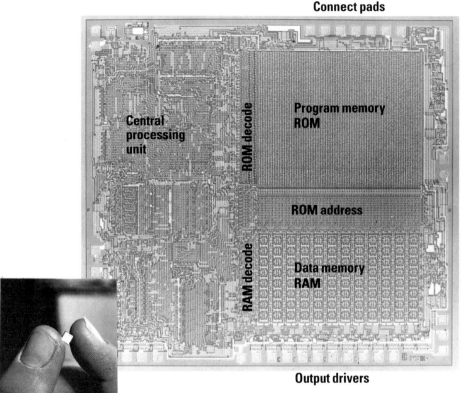

Connect pads

Central processing unit

ROM decode

Program memory ROM

Clock

ROM address

RAM decode

Data memory RAM

Clock driver circuit

Output drivers

The small computer in use

The circuity of a model 6500 microchip. This incorporates the 6502 microchip used in the Apple II. In effect, most of the central processing unit on the left of the 6500 is the 6502. The integration of the CPU, random access memory (RAM), read-only memory (ROM), clock and input/output drivers onto a single chip makes the 6500 a dedicated device, where the 6502 is general purpose.

In order for the computer to do anything it has to be programmed, a feature it shares with every general-purpose computer from the Analytical Engine onwards. The user may write programs specially for it, or make use of ready-written programs. Sometimes these come in the form of a written list or code, to be typed in via the keyboard. Often, though, programs are sold ready encoded onto a storage medium. The user simply slots in the read-only chip, disc or cassette encoded with the information, and tells the computer to read in the appropriate information.

What can the small computer do? In theory, it is general-purpose; in practice, it is limited by both its hardware and the operating instructions already encoded onto its chips. One important limitation is the languages in which it can be programmed; it will only understand languages that it has the facility to compile or interpret into its simple on/off code. This particular machine normally has the ability to run programs written in BASIC, PASCAL and COBOL. Each programming language has different strengths and weaknesses, but the instructions in all of them can be broken down into the simple manipulative operations discussed earlier.

A second major limitation lies in the amount of memory the computer has. It can only run programs that can be fitted into its capacity for data handling. And finally, it will be limited by its interfaces, the number of different input, output and communications devices to which it can be connected.

Within these limitations, though, the computer can do anything we can exhaustively tell it to do, in terms of its information-manipulative code. Throughout this book we will be describing computer applications, many of which can be carried out on microcomputers like the Apple II. You can probably add more to the list from your own dealings with computers at work, at home, in shops, banks, libraries, airports, and so on.

The dominating micro

Already computers and microprocessors, and the other technologies we have mentioned, are having a major impact upon our daily lives. The technological developments we have briefly outlined have brought us videophones, teleconferencing, modern methods of accountancy, forecasting, surveillance, and medical diagnosis and many other benefits (if that is the right word). There is virtually no area of our daily lives in which we cannot trace the influence of the silicon chip; indeed, there are few areas we do not mention at least in passing

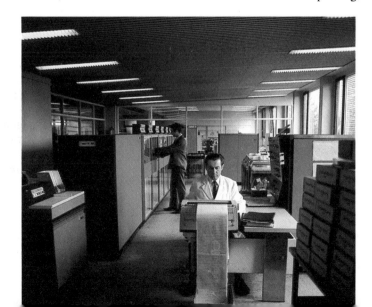

Centralized data processing: a mainframe computer used by the city of Düsseldorf in West Germany. A set-up like this relies on massive back-up storage on magnetic tape or hard disc.

in this book.

It is perhaps peculiar, then, that we should close this chapter by suggesting that the impact of the computer has been overestimated. It might be more accurate to say that by overestimating what the computer can do, we have allowed it to have an impact that is not appropriate to its great, but limited, capabilities.

We believe it is accurate to say that present-day computers, and other machines that use microelectronic circuits, might condition us to believe that they can shape our thinking. Perhaps they already have done so.

Many people speak of the computer as if it commands us, questions us and guides our thought. It is not always clear whether they mean these statements as metaphors. Even if they do, their repetition gives them an air of spurious authenticity and others may take them to be the literal truth. Perhaps simply by believing that the computer can shape their thoughts, these people do allow their thoughts to be shaped by the computer.

Yet there is little that is mysterious about computation as such. The basic add, subtract, compare and remember operations we have discussed are *all* that the computer can do. True, it can combine those operations in elaborate ways, and carry them out

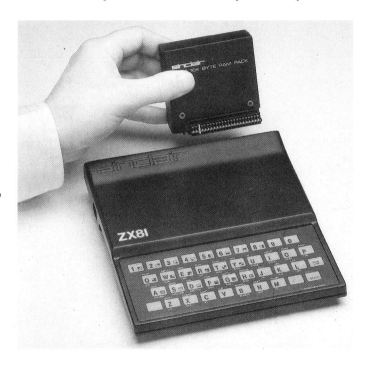

The Sinclair ZX81 pocket computer, launched in 1981, comes in ready-built or kit form and connects to a TV set or cassette recorder. Data or program storage can be multiplied 16 times by plugging an extra RAM unit into the back of the machine. The ZX 80, its predecessor, contained 21 separate chips; the ZX 81 has only four. Total cost, including a printer and RAM pack? Between £160 and £180 ($250 and $300).

at exceptional speed; but it cannot do anything *else*. Somehow, though, we persuade ourselves that the mysterious, the all-powerful computer *does* do something more.

This belief is encouraged by the use of simulations in which the computer is used to model specific real-life situations that can be anything from movements in the money supply to the flight of a jumbo jet. The accuracy of the simulation can be no better than the accuracy of the facts and assumptions from which the programmer worked, and of the program itself. But many people persuade themselves that because computer simulation is used as a tool in making predictions as to how a real-life situation will develop, the predictions that result are somehow more valid than predictions made without the aid of a computer. That is not necessarily the case. If the assumptions are poor, then the predictions based on them will be poor, however much computation is involved.

The situation becomes even more complex when the computer is used to simulate human thought processes. Research into artificial intelligence has succeeded in persuading the computer to simulate human thought. We look at some of the implications and consequences of this research later.

In the meantime, we might say that it is easy to look at a perfect (or even at a very good) imitation of thought and learning processes, of mind-like events, and take it for reality. If the computer converses with us in a way which even superficially resembles a conversation with another human being, we tend to forget that it is not necessarily thinking in a human way. But is *thinking* the right word to describe the process of computation?

That would perhaps be an easier question to answer if we had a better idea of how the human brain works and the nature of human thought processes. Can the computer think as a human being does? And if not, why not? What is there that is unique about the human brain, that makes it impossible for us to make the transition between saying that the computer simulates human thought, and saying that the computer thinks?

These are awkward questions. But in the age of micro man – in an age, that is, in which our world is full of microprocessors, and runs the risk of being dominated by them – they are questions we must consider.

Chapter 2 THE THREATENING COMPUTER

The scene: a factory that makes tubular steel chairs. A skilled painter is spraying a newly welded chair. He works economically and skillfully – up one leg, along the crossbar, down another leg – and the chair is evenly, perfectly painted. As he works a robot paint-sprayer attached to his arm follows his movements. When the chair is finished he stands back and another chair is placed in the same spot. The robot proceeds to paint it – up one leg, along the crossbar, down the next leg. The chair is just as evenly, just as perfectly painted.

Does this worry you? Before you reply, read this poem.

My head craves for joy
Blind to guilt perhaps calm
Seldom hoarding seldom aching
Passion if enforced
Destroys

It was written on a computer. A disturbing thought? Don't stop yet, though. Here is a newspaper report.

'Factory robot kills a worker. An industrial robot has killed a worker who was trying to repair it, the first accident of its kind in Japan, which has the world's largest robot work force. Details of the accident, which occurred in July at a plant of Kawasaki heavy industries, were revealed yesterday ... Kenji Urada, aged 37, a worker at the Akashi plant of the company, was trapped

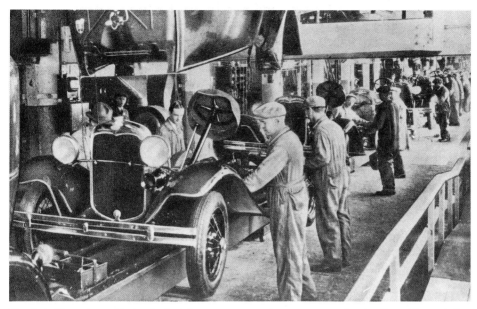

Nearly half a century of technological change separates these two car production lines. The cost of employing a human being on an assembly line today is twice or three times that of employing a robot, and the gap continues to widen.

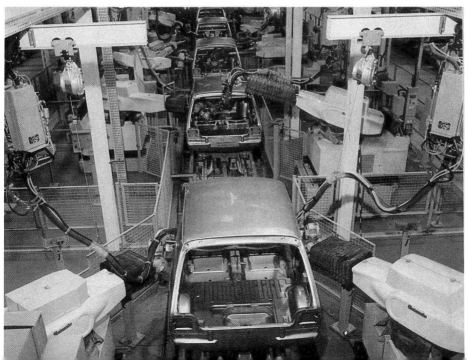

by the work arm of the robot which pinned him against a machine which cuts gears. He had enterd a prohibited area around the robot to repair it, the Labour Standards Bureau said. According to factory officials, a wire mesh fence around the robot would have shut off the unit's power supply when unhooked. But instead of opening it, Urada had apparently jumped over the fence. The employee set the machine on manual control but then accidentally brushed against the on switch, and the claw of the robot pushed him against the machine tooling device. Other workers were unable to stop the robot's action. Labour officials blamed a combination of unfamiliarity of the workers and neglect of regulations governing the new machines. The company said the robot had been removed from the line, and a man-high fence erected around two other robots working in the plant...'

Finally, something more down to earth. You reach the head of the Saturday morning line for the autobank machine, and put your card in the slot. The machine accepts your card, only to announce that it cannot process your request. You know your account should have money in it. You feel angry, embarrassed and powerless.

These are just four aspects of our relationship with computers that may irritate or even worry us. Is the worry justified? Is it simply caused by a lack of understanding of what computers are and what they do? We do not think so. Certainly anxiety has something to do with ignorance, but it is partly founded on the idea of threat – the belief that computers have minds of their own which are alien, if not actively hostile, to human values.

A robot can paint as well as a man, when it has been programmed to follow his movements. It cannot anticipate unforeseen circumstances such as no chair being put in place to be painted, but it will do a consistently efficient job in a fume-laden atmosphere which is unpleasant for human beings.

Can a computer write a poem? It can certainly be programmed to select words from its memory and assemble them in pre-determined ways. The programmer sets the parameters governing their assembly and the computer chooses, at random, the words that slot into those parameters. Do 'My head crave for joy ...' and the other poems reproduced opposite qualify as poetry or are they meaningless verse? Is a poem something that can only be written by a human being?

The robot did kill the man. But it did not do so maliciously or because it ran amok. It did so because the man broke the safety

MYSELF MANIFEST
Margaret Chisman, 1974

1st Selection

My head thrives on pain
Unseen by guilt
Not relaxing not seducing
Comfort if controlled
Corrupts

My eye quickens with grief
Bleak with doubt yet true
Rarely hoarding rarely aching
Sorrow if withheld
Consoles

My hand delights in rejection
Eager for despair ever calm
Beyond quarrelling beyond dreaming
Friendship if followed
Refreshes

My reason shades into enchantment
Strong with sin but dull
Above blaming above doubting
Freedom if enforced
Enslaves

My heart leads to caresses
Free from pride now soft
Sometimes probing sometimes pitying
Passion if enjoyed
Endures

My child craves for life
Free to lust never cruel
Seldom seeking seldom loving
Praise if derided
Destroys

My flesh yearns for joy
Ardent with dread perhaps fierce
Just hiding just daring
Remorse if applauded
Divides

My mood prepares for prayer
Blind to lies always vain
Only drifting only stifling
Truth if suppressed
Consumes

2nd Selection

My flesh leads to rejection
Free from despair never soft
Beyond hiding beyond dreaming
Remorse if applauded
Divides

My child thrives on grief
Ardent with pride yet true
Just seeking just dreaming
Truth if controlled
Corrupts

My heart quickens with enchantment
Eager for dread now fierce
Rarely blaming rarely seducing
Comfort if withheld
Enslaves

My hand shades into life
Unseen by sin always vague
Sometimes releasing sometimes stifling
Freedom if enjoyed
Refreshes

My reason delights in caresses
Bleak with lies maybe cruel
Not quarrelling not doubting
Friendship if derided
Consoles

My eye prepares for pain
Fresh to lust but vain
Above probing above loving
Praise if followed
Endures

My head craves for joy
Blind to guilt perhaps calm
Seldom hoarding seldom aching
Passion if enforced
Destroys

My mood yearns for prayer
Strong with doubt ever dull
Only drifting only pitying
Sorrow if suppressed
Consumes

regulations and got in the way of dangerous machinery. It was no more and no less dangerous than, say, a mechanical press. However, the story clearly inspired the journalist to make capital out of a common but irrational fear.

And the autobank machine? No, it had not withdrawn the last cent from your current account by mistake. It was simply telling you, in a tactless way, that your card was torn or bent. Tact was not programmed into it.

It is not so much what a computer does that annoys us or upsets us, but how it does it.

In the early days of electronic computing the human aspect received little attention. Those working with computers were scientists and engineers who expected the machinery they created to be awkward to handle and prone to maddening breakdowns and inexplicable pauses. Today a much wider population is obliged to interact with computers. We expect, indeed demand, 'user friendliness' – that the machine should present itself to us in useful and unforbidding guise. The computer industry has come some, though not all, of the way to meeting these requirements, but there are still many obstacles to 'computer friendliness'. Inexperienced users, for example, find it very difficult to re-order their natural language concepts and ways of thinking into computer language and computer logic. Suppose, for example, you want to ask a computer to find the average age of a large group of people. Your natural order of thinking is probably 'average', 'age' and people'; the computer might be programmed to receive commands only in the order 'average', 'people' and 'age'. The gap between you and the computer is trivial but it is real.

Getting on with computers

The most common response of skilled computer users to computers is exasperation. Broadly speaking the more user friendly a computer is, and the easier it is to gain access to processor time, the less exasperating it is to use. The frustrations of working with computers probably reached their height in the late 1960s and early 1970s, when commercial use was expanding rapidly. Computer time was still expensive and computers lacked the flexibility needed to meet a wide range of user requirements. Because of these limitations it was common for work on large mainframe computers to be scheduled on a batch

Stages in batch processing.

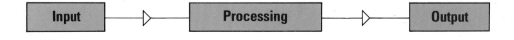

processing basis. In this process the user provides a 'batch' of input (typically a stack of punched cards), the computer processes it, and returns a stack of output (typically computer printout). The user need never see the computer; between the two come a host of operators and probably a few locked doors. The computer works fast, but getting the input to the computer, waiting for a slot in a heavy processing schedule, and getting the output back to the user may take anything from a day to a week. Air passengers may see a parallel in the ratio of time taken up actually flying and time spent in the departure lounge. Although batch processing is still used for some slow-moving and large commercial operations the longueurs involved make it impractical for many jobs.

The more usual processing method today is an interactive one, in which the central processor is directly available to users via terminals. In local networks the terminals are connected by cables to the central processor; alternatively, the terminal may be coupled to the processor via direct-dial telephone lines. Terminal and computer are coupled throughout the processing operation, and the computer can output data or request further input, and receive data or new instructions, while a program is being run.

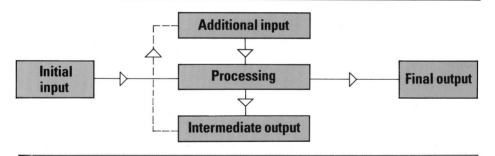

Stages in interactive processing.

Terminals can be used for batch input as well; the user types in a batch of data that is then transmitted directly to the central processor, or stored by the terminal's own microprocessor and transmitted later, perhaps at an off-peak time. The central processor gets to work and at the end of the processing returns the output to the terminal.

'Time sharing' systems enable many user terminals to be linked to the same central processor. Such systems, however, are very sensitive to overload, and when processing time was expensive many systems were often loaded up to or above their limits. As a result, frustrated users had to wait for access for seconds, minutes, or even hours, rather than the scarcely perceptible interval intended by the designer.

Today such delays are rarer. Many terminals now contain their own local processing facilities, easing the burden on the central processor which need only be called upon for stored data or more complex programs. But the ludicrous still occurs. At peak hours in the University of Naples you may have to wait five to fifteen minutes for the central time-shared system to draw the co-ordinates of a graph. On an equivalent machine dedicated to one user this would take milliseconds.

Exasperation can be further compounded if there are lengthy communication lines between the terminal and central processor. A typical example is that of a computer with specialized programs being used by a far-flung clientèle. Delays occur because the communication lines consist of several portions, all of which must become available at the same time. P L A T O , a well-known system for computer-aided learning, used to take minutes before its main machine in Brussels would respond with the start of a tutorial.

We find similar problems with large database systems offering access to a wide range of information, either to the general public (via the telephone system) or to a large but distinct user group (all the branches of a bank, for instance). It is not easy to structure databases so that all the information they contain is easily accessible. Thick user manuals are off-putting, and long searches through the data bank are expensive and time-consuming. Prestel, the British Telecom viewdata system, uses a combination of a user directory and a tree information structure with an index that leads the user to information 'pages'. However, recent surveys have shown that even regular users are not particularly successful in tracking down the information they want. In a typical hunt through the database a user will have to access five pages before reaching the one he or she wants. Only about 60 per cent of Prestel's predominantly business users manage to do so successfully.

With the advent of low-priced microprocessors powerful enough to run all the but the largest applications many of the problems of batch processing and time sharing are fading. But experience with viewdata systems suggests that new problems are taking their place. As computing ability expands, so do our ambitions. Even today user requirements often seem to come second to technical requirements in designing new systems. All too often computer codes, look-up search techniques and programming facilities are technically easy to implement but, in human terms, perverse to use.

**The ethical
boundaries
of computers**

If the computer is exasperating rather than frightening to trained computer users, it can be both exasperating and frightening to researchers in artificial intelligence. To them the computer is far more than a calculating machine. It is, in effect, the tool with which they attempt to reproduce a wide range of intelligent behaviour.

Scientists in general are notoriously unaware of the moral and social implications of their work. However researchers into artificial intelligence have a powerful critic in their ranks in the person of Joseph Weizenbaum of the Massachusetts Institute of Technology. His critique of artificial intelligence and its wider implications, *Computer Power and Human Reason*, was published in 1976.

Weizenbaum accepts that if artificial intelligence research is pursued far enough it may be possible to design machines for use in areas that are currently regarded as exclusively human, areas that involve many types of thought other than the purely logical-deductive. If this is the case, where should we draw the line between machine work and human work so as to leave a distinctive role for ourselves? Certain types of activity must be designated as human, not to be performed by machines. Artificial intelligence research in these areas should be discouraged; there is plenty for researchers to do elsewhere.

Which areas should be taboo? Fundamentally, those that involve interpersonal understanding. Weizenbaum takes as an example his own program ELIZA, that simulates, albeit in a simplistic way, the responses of a Rogerian psychotherapist. The essence of Rogerian or client-centred therapy is that the therapist adopts a non-judgemental, empathic and positive attitude towards clients and their problems. ELIZA does not make any attempt to understand the client's emotions or moral dilemmas but it does provide responses appropriate enough to sustain a dialogue. For instance:

> **Patient** I am very depressed.
>
> ELIZA I am sorry to hear you are depressed.
>
> **Patient** I blame my parents.
>
> ELIZA Tell me more about your parents.

Simple though the program is, conversation with ELIZA proved sufficiently involving for a host of people to beg to 'talk' to the computer. Weizenbaum rebelled. It is not desirable, he argued, for people to delude themselves that they are getting psychiatric help when they are merely responding to a computer program. Psychotherapy demands the sympathetic involvement

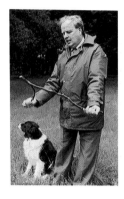

Water divining, a valued skill even in the age of micro man. Oil prospecting, however, is being computerized, so huge are the rewards of finding oil.

A case of the tail wagging the dog? Technological exuberance aside, there is a need to clearly formulate where the boundaries between humans and computers lie. Because a machine can replace a man, must it?

of a fellow human being, and for a machine to aspire to give that involvement (and it was sugested that a refined version of ELIZA might do so) is obscene.

Weizenbaum's book has been criticized at length, with humanity and thoughtfulness, by others in the field of artificial intelligence. Little common ground has emerged. Weizenbaum, for instance, finds it an appalling thought that a machine should be coupled up to an animal's brain in the hope of learning something useful. Others, after long and careful thought, fail to find the idea appalling. Since Weizenbaum's argument in this case is based primarily on emotion, no reconciliation between the two views is possible. Either you feel horror or you do not.

Perhaps the most intriguing question, though, is what programs like ELIZA actually do. As attempts at teaching a computer to converse they are primitive. Nevertheless they do involve interactions with human beings. Are those people who believe, mistakenly, that the computer 'understands' them, also deluding themselves that they are being helped? Or is ELIZA, by directing their thoughts along tangential paths, helping them to articulate and re-think their problems? If it really does help them, irrespective of how it does so, is it wrong to refuse them that help?

A similar issue arises in connection with computer art. What is art? To many people an essential part of a work of art is knowing or believing that it is an attempt by another human being to communicate ideas, or emotions, or sensations. Even a blank canvas on a gallery wall is not the same as a blank canvas in an art supplies shop. The artist's decision to show the untouched canvas as a work of art imbues it with meaning.

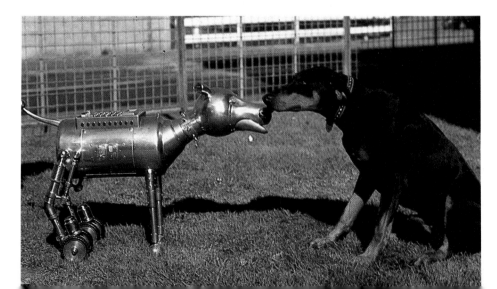

If art is defined as human-to-human communication, a verse by a computer is not a poem. To present a verse written by a computer as if it were a poem written by a human being is a fraud, just as it is a fraud to submit an 'abstract painting' by a monkey to an art exhibition. But Margaret Chisman's poems (see page 35) are not truly 'computer verse'; she is using the computer as a tool to write her own poems. And the same is true of today's computer-generated visual art. The part the computer plays in producing it is minimal compared with the choices made by the programmer-artist.

Should we insist that computers of the future remain tools? Our view is that if we do, we shall deny ourselves some hugely enriching possibilities.

Techno fear

Many people find technology, especially computer technology, intimidating. The purposeful robot is a potent symbol of this techno fear. Why should this be? Even though today's factory robots are not even remotely humanoid, an anthropomorphic image of robots persists, cultivated by generations of science fiction books and films. The Golem of middle-European Jewish folklore, Frankenstein's monster, the zombies or living dead of voodoo myth are all cultural archetypes of the mechanical man without human feelings. In a persistent nightmare the robot advances on us implacably, with neither pity nor hatred, to crush us, strangle us with superhuman and impartial strength. It is an image of hopelessness in which there can be no appeal to human values of warmth, compassion, generosity or humour.

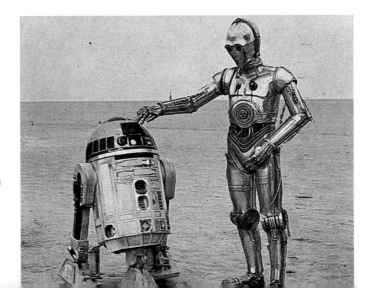

R2D2 and C3P0 from Star Wars, great favourites with millions of children. Is this because they have qualities that no computer yet possesses?

To keep this fear at bay, the science fiction writer Isaac Asimov invented three rules of robotics, a neat set of moral guidelines for the control of robotic behaviour. These state:

1.   A robot may not attack a human being or, through inaction, allow a human being to come to harm.

2.   A robot must obey the orders given it by a human being except where such orders would conflict with the first law.

3.   A robot must protect its own existence as long as such protection does not conflict with the first and second laws.

However, as Marvin Minsky, Professor of Mathematics and Computer Science at Massachusetts Institute of Technology, has pointed out, we are a long way from learning how to instil such guidelines into microprocessors. How is a microprocessor to recognize a human? How is it to recognize the concept of harm? Long before we have solved these problems we may be saddled with complex machines and populations of machines, with many layers of interleaved programs, which we do not fully understand and cannot fully control. Minsky admits that there is a possibility that the first generation of smart machines may be psychotic. True, we may learn to make robots sane and well-adjusted in time, but until we do we could be in for an uncomfortable few years. Perhaps the only sensible course is to treat computers as we treat our fellow human beings, and work on the assumption that they mean us no harm until the opposite is proven.

There are grounds for optimism. Our experience so far tells us that a reasonably well designed computer system makes a complex process which has to be kept within strict limits safer than it would be if it were controlled by a human alone. Of course computers can break down and programs can exhibit unforeseen bugs. But human beings are even less trustworthy; their attention wanders, they like to think all is well when it manifestly is not, and they react slowly and irrationally in moments of crisis.

The risk inherent in the optimistic view is that we may place too much confidence in the infallibility of computers. We entrust them with the control of processes – such as those involved in nuclear reactors – which we would not dream of setting up if we ourselves had to control them. Even the most foolproof safety precautions may be wrecked by a random malfunction.

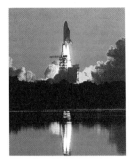

Lift-off for the Columbia space shuttle. The systems that guide vehicles in space also target missiles on earth.

Does this mean that we should be more afraid of computers as controllers than of computers as calculators? Certainly, the outcome of an error in a computer controlling a nuclear power plant could be disastrous. But a human decision based on a calculating error, or on a calculation which is correct but based on false premises, could be equally disastrous. An alarming example of this occurred in June 1980 when a computer malfunction caused the North American Air Defense Command to think that Soviet missiles had been fired at the United States; a full-scale retaliatory alert was instigated.

To most people, however, Armageddon is a more distant worry than the immediate threat of redundancy. Many people are understandably worried about their skills becoming progressively less attractive, because uneconomical, to their employers. Are computers stealing our jobs?

Computers and jobs

Unemployment has less to do with the impact of microtechnology than with industry's lack of long-term plans to meet foreign competition, complacency in the face of new technology, and poor marketing and distribution.

It is not easy to measure the impact of microprocessors on jobs because so many other economic and human factors are involved. In the 1960s and early 1970s industries that automated were generally expanding anyway, and changes in job patterns caused few tremors. Recessions are influenced only marginally by the impact of new technology. Firms that are faring badly do not invest in microprocessor-controlled machinery, while firms that do invest appear to do comparatively well. Not surprisingly trade unions tend to see investment as a hopeful sign, and though they negotiate to safeguard

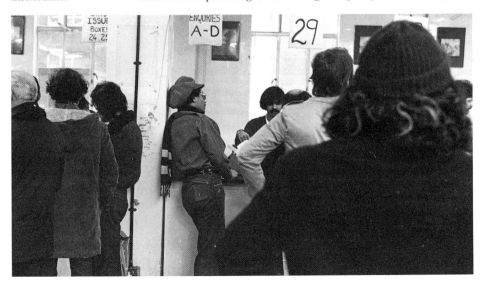

their members' interests, they rarely discourage such investment. Firms that invest in advanced technology are firms that
are confident about the future.

All the same it is only common sense to assume that as
investment in computer technology goes up, so must productivity per employee. If it does not, something is drastically
wrong. Does this mean a shrinking, if more productive, work
force? Not necessarily. Jobs do not have to be lost as a direct
result of new technology. The alternatives include producing
more goods at less cost and expanding markets, producing
better goods that sell in greater numbers or at higher prices, or
exploring new product areas opened up by the new technology
itself. It is along these lines that progressive companies, unions
and governments usually think.

A recent OECD (Organization for Economic Co-operation
and Development) survey of the predicted effect of microelectronics on employment, *Microelectronics, Productivity
and Employment*, included some revealing figures from Japan.
Jobs in Japanese industry, it says, will reduce by between
200 000 and 500 000 as a result of the introduction of
microelectronics, but by the same token some 700 000 additional jobs, all computer-related, will be created. So although
not all redundant production line workers will immediately
re-train to fill computer maintenance or programming jobs, the
total numbers of jobs in industry could increase.

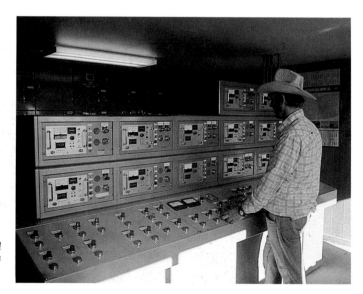

A 'computer cowboy'
operates a sophisticated
feed-mix installation on
a cattle ranch in
Alberta, Canada.

Caxton's printing press put an end to the illuminated manuscript industry. Now, 500 years later, computer setting is replacing hand setting of type for most commercial purposes. A whole page of type can be reset in a different face or to a different size at the touch of a button.

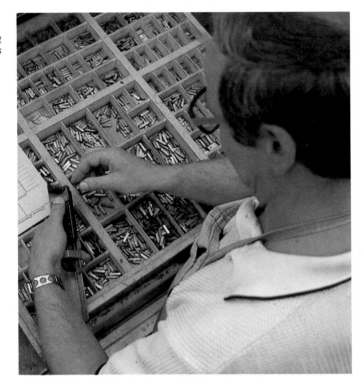

In the long run it seems certain that we will evolve new life styles and patterns of employment – flexible work hours and fewer of them, more frequent re-training, more integration of home and family life – to suit the microchip age. Before the first Industrial Revolution people would have been amazed and appalled to hear that in 1981 only about 2 per cent of the United States work force would be engaged in agriculture. 'What does the other 98 per cent do?' they would have asked. When manufacturing industries are fully automated, offices are crammed with word processors and terminals, and shopping is done by remote ordering from unmanned warehouses, what will the people of the year 2100 do? We suggest that they may have time to be more human, and time to pursue the interests that once got squeezed into the small interstices between work and family.

Working with machines need not mean less enjoyable work. It does not follow that because one works with a machine one becomes a dehumanized component of it. Dehumaniz-ation merely reflects poor or exploitative management, or poor social policies. Technological changes, whether they lead to fewer jobs or to different jobs, must be handled in ways that cause least human distress. There is absolutely no doubt, however, that in a microprocessor-controlled world a vast amount of dirty, unhealthy and boring work will be done by machines.

Cultural and spiritual values

There is another aspect to techno fear, however, more insidious than that aroused by the prospect of changes in work patterns. This is the fear of 'mental castration', fear of being outdone in those areas in which we most pride ourselves. Indeed the process is already under way. Most insurance salesmen today can neither add nor multiply adeptly, the supermarket cash till requires little acumen, and how many people regularly write letters? The clerical skills of the past century – such as keeping a handwritten ledger, or the ability to write business letters in copperplate – are already disappearing from our culture just as the chivalries and courtesies of earlier ages have vanished forever.

Another fear is that learning, and the imaginative use of what we learn, will become redundant. What will be the point of acquiring knowledge when any database contains a million times more accessible information than our brain? Why try to use personally acquired knowledge when a computer can apply it more efficiently, more appropriately? Perhaps all that we now think of as knowledge will come to seem sterile and pointless to future generations.

At its most acute, mental castration might lead to a total loss of feelings of individual identity and worth. If and when machines can emulate and even surpass us in every measurable area of human endeavour, what uniquely human pursuits will be left to us?

Computers are undeniably superior to humans in the speed and efficiency with which they calculate, in the manipulation of colours, graphics and perspective, and in their ability to store facts. They are also superior in certain aspects of problem solving. Nevertheless it will be many years before we create machines with the common sense of a child of five. What forms of work are we prepared to entrust to a child of five, always recognizing of course that a lot of work requires less intelligence than that of a child of five?

We have lived with machines for generations, but we have emotional and spiritual resources that have prevented us from becoming obsessed with them. Most of us can pass by a Space Invaders machine without an agonizing inner struggle. There

Right:
Mozambique, 1977.
None of the atrocities of this or any other century has been committed by computer. Yet computer power is helping us to multiply the range and scale of our weapons of destruction.

Inset: Information overload?

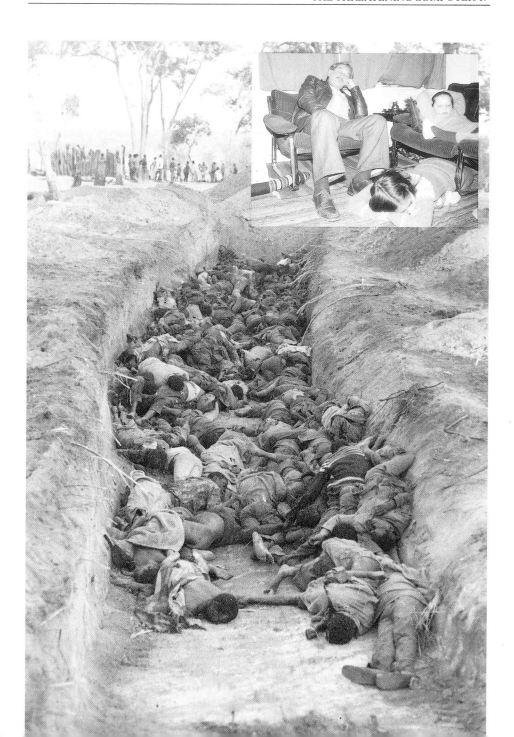

'If all your humanoids are destroyed, then the planet surface disappears and all the invaders turn into mutants which mount a sustained attack on your craft' (quote from a computer games article). How closely do players identify with zapping aliens, nuking monsters and blowing planets to dust? Many amusement arcade games like Space Invaders and its descendants are now available on home computers.

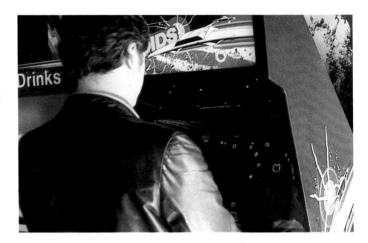

is, we believe, a limit to the effects which computers will have on our civilization and culture. Already the machine age has spawned its counter-revolutionaries. The emergence of beatniks, flower children, fringe religions, environmental lobbies, craft revivals, new spectator sports – all assert the force of values that are impervious to the onslaught of technology.

The threat to privacy

Much concern has been expressed about the erosion of privacy in modern, highly regulated information societies. When interactive cable television becomes the norm, for example, it will be all too easy for government and private agencies to find out about our political opinions, our buying habits, our family and friends, our financial status, our leisure activities. As fast as information networks are being devised security systems are being developed to regulate the leakage or dissemination of information. The code makers and the code breakers are running a race in which the makers never edge more than marginally ahead. Most of us feel more strongly about personal than institutional privacy, insisting on the right to know but wishing to limit the right to be known. There has always been a fundamental conflict between freedom of information and confidentiality. A computerized society will take us deeper into that conflict than ever before, but there are some safeguards in computer-information networks that did not exist in their more fallible and chaotic predecessors. Most computerized credit information services today give individuals the right to inspect their own credit records and to put right any wrong information contained in them. With the old systems it was not possible to do this.

Followers of the
Bhagwan Shree
Rajneesh. A recent
Bhagwan
advertisement offers
meditation, Sufi
dancing and
experiential workshops
... with video tuition.
Clearly spiritual values
and new technology are
quite compatible.

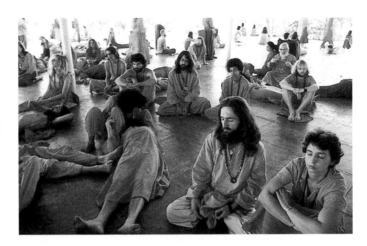

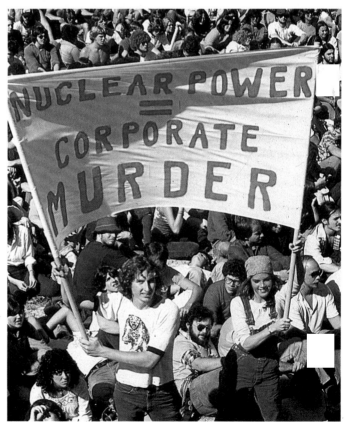

Anti-nuclear
demonstrators in the
United States. Asserting
the values of a past age,
or values proper to the
age of the computer?

Also, the very fact that decision procedures in computer programs have to be spelled out clearly and exhaustively to some extent prevents human prejudices being incorporated into them. Although a human user can be biased and feed in biased information, the computer itself is not biased, not prejudiced against the old, the young, or racial minorities. A computerized system is a system in which fallible human judgement is replaced by decisions made according to generally fair rules.

As the computer takes over the clerical chores that underpin so much of the structure of government, it seems likely that humans may have more time to indulge in human compassion and understanding. Will we have civil servants, in the year 2100, who are unharassed and take a real interest in the problems and suggestions of their client public? Will the systems they administer fit the needs of the public rather than the constraints of their staffs?

Computer systems never get harassed. They can politely and unhurriedly conduct essential but repetitive interviews with hospital patients, job hunters or people claiming social benefits. Pilot studies done in the United Kingdom, in the cities of Brighton and Cardiff, used a program which asked claimants about their circumstances and on the basis of their answers suggested which benefits they might be entitled to.

Unauthorized interference

In many ways the information systems of tomorrow will be less prone to fraud and sabotage than those of today. The simple net or ring structure outlined in Chapter 3 is vulnerable to deliberate disruption as well as breakdown, but as the interconnections become more complex, as systems come to incorporate more redundant components, and as control becomes a shifting and adaptable function, so the ability of a given system to cope with unauthorized interference becomes greater.

An example of such interference, and its limitations, is the recent phenomenon of computer crime. This category of crime has undoubtedly grown along with the numbers of computers, but the picture is complicated by the reluctance of defrauded companies to prosecute – less than one in ten do so according to some estimates. Don Parker of the Stanford Research Institute, California, has estimated that financial loss was a factor in 324 of the 669 known cases of computer abuse in the United States in the years 1958 to 1969. Those 324 cases accounted for total losses of $546 million.

Yet many of the computer frauds in the 1950s and 1960s

Computer fraud in the United Kingdom

Type of Fraud	Number of Frauds	Value of Loss (£)	($)
Unauthorized alteration of input	42	858 170	1 550 000
Misappropriation of output	2	3 600	6 500
Misuse of programs	1	26 000	47 000
Misuse of computer time/resources	22	17 379	31 300
Total	67	905 149	1 634 800

(Source: Local Government Audit Inspectorate, quoted in Computerworld UK, 2 September 1981)

were extremely simple. Relying on management ignorance and on inadequate audit procedures, personnel with access to the computer simply milked accounts of stray cents, or added fictitious names to the payroll. Opportunities for doing this are much rarer now that security precautions are tighter. Nevertheless a major banking development, the electronic transfer of funds, has been seriously delayed by the need to develop adequate security precautions.

What people think about computers

In 1971 Time magazine and the American Federation of Information Processing Societies carried out a major survey of public attitudes to computers in the United States. The 1 001 interviews, conducted with a statistically selected sample of the adult population, highlighted a number of fears and doubts about the impact of computers. There has been no comparable survey since, but small soundings made in recent years suggest that attitudes have remained fairly stable.

On the whole respondents were fairly clear about what computers could and could not do; they believed that computers cannot think for themselves, and that computers of the future would not disobey the instructions of the people running them. Nevertheless there was plenty of anxiety about unwanted surveillance and snooping, about job security, about over-dependency on computers. A majority thought that computers would increase leisure time, make government more effective and reduce the chances of war. The majority also thought that many of the current uses of computers should be increased, except for the purposes of advertising and dating.

There was, perhaps, too much willingness to entrust decisions about proper and improper computer use to the government. We believe that it is essential for every concerned

Attitudes to the computer. Total sample 1 001. A Time magazine/AFIPS survey.

	Agree	Percentage of total sample	
		Don't know/ No answer	Disagree
The development of large computerized information files will help make our government more effective	63	8	29
Computers will be used to keep people under surveillance	58	7	35
Safeguards are used by the government to make sure that personal information stored in computers is accurate	53	19	28
The government will determine what computers can and connot be used for	57	9	34
Computers create more jobs than they eliminate	36	13	51
Because of computerized information files, too many people have information about other people	58	9	33
Computers represent a real threat to people's privacy	38	8	54
Computerized information files may be used to destroy individual freedom	53	7	40
People are becoming too dependent on computers	55	7	38
Computers are more reliable than people	49	8	43
There is no way to find out if the information about you that is stored in a computer is accurate	42	14	44
'Computer mistakes' are really mistakes made by people who use computers	81	6	13
Computers can produce results that are more accurate than the information they are given	30	13	57
The use of computers increases the chance of war	17	13	70
Computers will create more leisure time for people	86	2	12
Computers are dehumanizing people and turning them into numbers	54	6	40
Computers of the future might disobey the instructions of the people who run them	23	8	69
Computers can think for themselves	12	5	83

citizen of the modern world to understand the computer environment that is taking shape, and to understand it well enough to play some part in shaping it. The high proportion of 'Don't knows' in the second part of the survey presumably reflected ignorance – 'I don't know enough about computers to have an opinion'.

It is not the computer itself which should give us cause for concern but the ways in which we use it. The computer is still a machine that only adds, subtracts and compares.

From the same survey, answers to the question: 'The following uses of the computer should be increased or decreased?'

	Increase	Don't know/ No answer	Decrease
Keeping track of criminals	78	16	6
Gathering and analyzing census data	70	24	6
Medical diagnosis	74	15	11
Guidance of missiles for national defense	71	18	11
Vote counting	66	26	8
Credit card billing systems	52	35	13
Surveillance of activist or radical groups	56	27	17
Automatic control of factory machinery	53	31	16
Credit card reference checks	52	31	17
Projection of election results based on early voting returns	50	30	20
Public opinion polling	47	34	19
Compiling information files on US citizens	50	24	26
Teaching children in school	48	27	25
Matching of people for dating	14	31	55
Sending mail advertisements to the home	16	21	63

How should we use the computer then? Do we want it to rival the power and sophistication of our own minds, or do we merely want to increase its block-busting, number-crunching power? Do we want it to take over all work, or only some work?

Chapter **3 COMPUTERS, CONSCIOUSNESS & CONFLICT**

Intelligent Beermats.
*Normally covered with
a writing surface, these
modules can be
re-arranged in any
order to give a computer
alternative ground
plans of a building. John
Frazer of Ulster
Polytechnic (Northern
Ireland) developed this
idea after seeing an
architect in a bar
sketching on beer
coasters.*

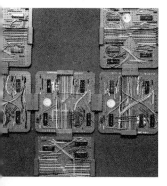

Can a computer think? Can it be intelligent? Of course not, you may say, and many experts on computing will probably agree with you. However, others argue that computers have always 'thought', albeit in a very limited way, and that today the range of ways in which they can think, and the depth of their intelligence, is growing dramatically.

The study of artificial intelligence, or the display of intelligent behaviour by non-living things, is still controversial. Many intelligence researchers complain that 'intelligence' is defined by their critics as being what computers cannot yet display. Perhaps this is true, but defining intelligence and thought is not straightforward. You have to think about whether thinking necessarily involves a living being, and even whether a computer might not be a living being in some sense.

One common definition is that computers can be said to think if they perform tasks that would require thought if you did them yourself. The arithmetic and logic operations of conventional computers can be put into this category. In this sense computers think, even though they only carry out the instructions in their program. Their arithmetic and logic operations are akin to logical deduction. But deduction is only one form of thought. What of induction, of reasoning by analogy, of making hypotheses, of asking questions, of innovation and creativity? Although it would seem rather ridiculous to have asked whether Babbage's Analytical Engine or even a 1940s computer could think creatively, it is by no means a ridiculous question to ask about some of the computer networks of today. Somehow it no longer seems to be so obviously and inevitably true that computers cannot create, cannot hypothesize, cannot hold a conversation with us.

The rise of the computer network

The concept of the stored program was essential to the development of the time dimension of computing. It led to the realization that it was possible to divorce the timescale of input from that of computation proper, and these in turn from that of output. First the computer could receive all the input necessary for it to run a particular program; then it would execute the program; and then it would output the results. It was relatively immaterial whether the speed of input and output was comparable to the speed of processing or not. As a result, computers developed to work at faster and faster processing speeds, while input and output operations were still conducted at speeds which allowed for the slower reactions of human beings.

For many programs, however, this linear time process – input, processing, output – is not an adequate schematic. With the emergence of 'user friendly' input and output devices– terminals with keyboard and video display units, on which it was quicker and simpler to communicate with the computer – came the development of interactive programming. An interactive program enables the computer to appear to conduct a conversation with the operator. It asks for, and receives, fresh input (data or instructions) during the actual processing operation. But the increasing disparity between computer response time and human response time meant that the processor waited idly during each input phase for what were, by computer time standards, long periods. Similarly, the need to output results, or requests for further input, during the execution of the program also led to stretches of idle processing time.

Human response time was not the only culprit. Computer keyboards and printers, and data storage devices such as magnetic tape and punched cards, all operate more slowly than the central processor.

The cost of computing in the 1960s and early 1970s was such that it was desirable to use the processor as fully as possible. As a result, operating procedures were developed to circumvent this kind of impasse. It became common for computers to handle several different programs at once. Data for one program might be input while another program was being run. The computer might simultaneously output data from one program on a slow printer, and data from another on a video display unit. It might even carry out processing steps from several different programs alternately.

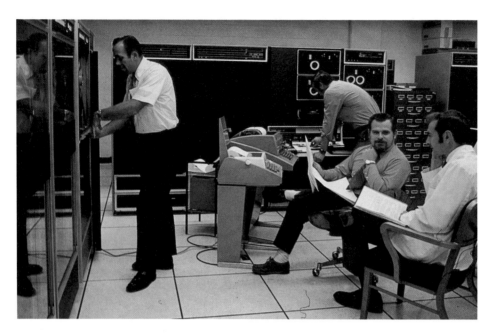

Clinicians and laboratory technicians using the expensive resources of a central processor on a time sharing basis.

An executive program inside the computer handled the flow of traffic. From time to time it would initiate a search to discover which components were in use, or available for use. In this way the most serious bottlenecks were eliminated.

The time sharing practices of this era, when it was standard for many users to make use of the same central processor, are far less common today. Indeed they led the computer industry up something of a blind alley. The decreasing cost of processing power brought about by microelectronics meant that it was no longer necessary to utilize processors so intensively, and today's mini and micro computers do not generally possess the complex executive programs that characterized the previous generation of mainframe computers.

The executive program was superseded by the general resource allocation supervisor, designed to predict the availability of components and make the best possible use of free components. As the system of networked components controlled by this type of device became more complex, it became practicable to introduce additional processors into the system. Nowadays, it is common to find machine architectures which use several central processing units. Probably the earliest operational machines to do so were Illiac 3 and 4, developed at the University of Illinois.

The most obvious advantage of linking machines together, or of incorporating several microprocessors into a single machine, is that the resulting configuration is faster and more convenient to program and use.

However, using not one but several processors leads to a major change of emphasis. When a system contains only one processing unit, it can carry out only one processing operation at a time – one act of addition, subtraction or comparison on one set of data. Though the speed at which such operations are carried out is now unimaginable – up to three million or more operations per second – the computer still has to be programmed so that operations are performed strictly one at a time.

Incorporating more than one processor in a system introduces the possibility of carrying out more than one act of addition, subtraction or comparison at a time, and handling more than one set of data at a time. This is usually called 'parallel computation'.

In a system that is running several programs simultaneously, parallel acts of computation may all relate to different programs. The advantages of the system are more practical than conceptual. It is also possible, in some types of system, to use the technique of parallel computation within the confines of a single program.

Computer networks and parallel processing

However elaborately they are combined, the components of present-day computer networks are still essentially those described earlier – input devices, memory devices, controllers, arithmetic logic units, and output devices. The circuits of computer networks are still made up of the same on-off transistors and other basic electronic components.

It is largely a matter of convenience whether the components of a computer system are housed in one box or widely separated. If the users of the system are themselves dispersed, then separation – given an efficient communications network – is much more cost-effective than concentration. An agglomeration of microprocessors and peripheral devices can be linked together in many ways, including 'nets' and 'rings.'

A typical example of a net is shown opposite. In this arrangement there is one centralized controller, usually itself a microprocessor, a number of other microprocessors, and input, output and storage devices. A particular microprocessor will have the peripheral devices it uses most at its own location, but it will also have access to other components in the network for less frequent or more specialized jobs. Messages, which may be data or instructions, are routed through the central controller to the microprocessors, each of which deals with its own computation

Plan of a typical microprocessor net.

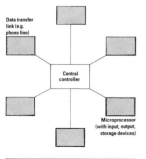

Data transfer link (e.g. phone line)

Central controller

Microprocessor (with input, output, storage devices)

separately, co-ordinated by the timing of the controller. With several microprocessors in the net, there will be several operations going on during each interval counted by the controlling clock. This is a form of parallel operation, but with no direct interaction between the different operations being performed simultaneously. Program steps are linked together in time only.

The drawing below shows a ring, a loop-like organization of connected computers (again including some with special capabilities). In this ring structure messages are handled by sending them round the ring as 'packets' with 'labels' on them. The labels describe the functional capabilities needed to handle the messages to which they are attached. A package circulates until a suitable processor is free, the function indicated by the label is performed, and the result is sent to the return address indicated on the packet.

The advantages that rings and nets offer over disconnected microcomputers are purely practical. Users have extensive computing resources immediately available at their own locations and will normally be able to treat them as personal. However, when additional resources are needed, they borrow them from elsewhere in the network, just as their resources may be borrowed by others. The resources in question might be hardware (a faster or better quality printer) or software (a specialized editing program). Together these hardware and software resources give the aggregation of machines in the net or ring much of the power and sophistication of a large mainframe computer.

Although a single centralized computer still has advantages for some applications, where data must be up-to-the-minute or where very complex scientific calculations are required, a network of small microprocessors is often more flexible. Programs need not be co-ordinated as closely, which makes for easier programming and faster operation. This type of architecture is now well established. New microprocessor network systems are announced at frequent intervals, and at least half of those launched prove commercially viable.

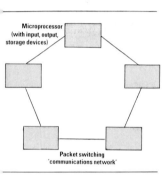

Microprocessor (with input, output, storage devices)

Packet switching 'communications network'

Plan of a typical microprocessor ring.

Expert systems

Expert systems are closely related to microprocessor networks of the kind just described. An expert system is one which attempts to harness the knowledge of human experts in a particular field – in medicine or geology for example – to computer processing power. An expert system is designed to solve problems that demand thought plus a huge fund of background knowledge.

The machines that go to make up an expert system are

The human expert at work, measuring a patient's blood pressure with a sphygmomanometer. The mercury gauge of the sphygmomanometer registers the pressure transmitted along the surface artery each time the heart beats, and also the pressure between heart beats.

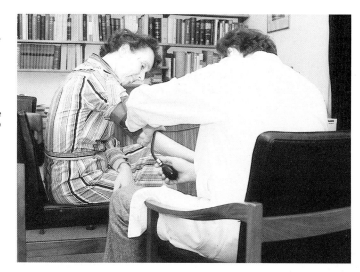

programmed to perform specific tasks, to act as 'specialists'. They are provided with specialist data or are programmed to carry out specialist procedures, and the data fed into them and the special procedures they carry out are adapted to the problem in hand.

There are several methods of controlling the way in which an expert system handles a problem. The problem can be divided into its constituent parts, and each part dealt with by the appropriate specialist machine. There is no collaboration between the machines during the different processing operations. Another method is to program the expert system to subdivide the problem itself. The different parts of the problem are then delegated to the appropriate specialist machine. There is, in this arrangement, a sense in which the parallel processing performed by the system is interactive. However, the interaction is fixed by the programmer. It does not lead to any real enhancement of the system's 'thinking' power.

Array processors

An entirely different form of parallel processing takes place in an array processor. In this case, the parallel operations occur within one special-purpose device, and not in a network (though it would of course be feasible to include an array processor as a special feature in a net or ring).

In a serial computer, the arithmetic/logic unit handles only two pieces of data at once. Let us describe its action by a very simple schematic. Imagine that the machine has two 'active' locations, A and B. The control unit ensures that two designated pieces of data are deposited in A and B, and the arithmetic/logic unit then performs tasks such as:

adding the data in A to the data in B;

subtracting the data in A from the data in B;

comparing the data in A and B, according to some fixed criterion.

It is possible to program virtually all arithmetic/logic based processing tasks so that they can be performed in this serial manner: by carrying out an arithmetic/logic operation on only two pieces of data at once, and repeating the operation as often as necessary on different data. But this is not always the most efficient way of handling problems. In particular, pattern recognition (recognizing a specific component from a selection of nuts and bolts, or distinguishing the letter 'b' from the letter 'd', for instance) is extremely cumbersome approached in this way.

An array processor solves the problem by exchanging our two locations, A and B, for an array of locations, for a number of different locations arranged in a fixed pattern. In practice array of locations are designed in three or more dimensions, but for the moment let us imagine a two-dimensional array of 35 locations arranged in 5 rows and 7 columns, as shown below.

We will indicate how the array processor works by suggesting briefly (and in a very simplified way) how it might go about recognizing, say, the letter A. It will have in its memory the concept of how the letter A is made up, a set of alternative patterns all of which it will interpret as being A. These will be stored in an on-off, or black-white (essentially the same) array, as shown below.

A simple 5 x 7 array of storage locations, and three alternative ways of storing the letter A in a 5 x 7 array. An array processor would recognize any of these patterns as A.

When the processor is given a pattern to interpret, it will divide it into squares matching the locations in its array pattern, and then look simultaneously at each square to see if its contents match those of the equivalent square in a pattern in its memory. If all the squares match, or nearly so, it will recognize the pattern as being the same as one its memory, in this case as an A.

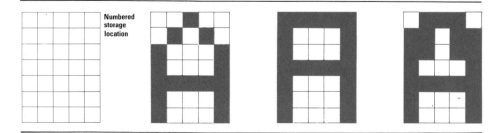

Numbered storage location

This satellite map of the Persian Gulf has been computer-enhanced to increase contrast between the salient features of the area. Enhanced images give less information but they give you the information that is important to you.

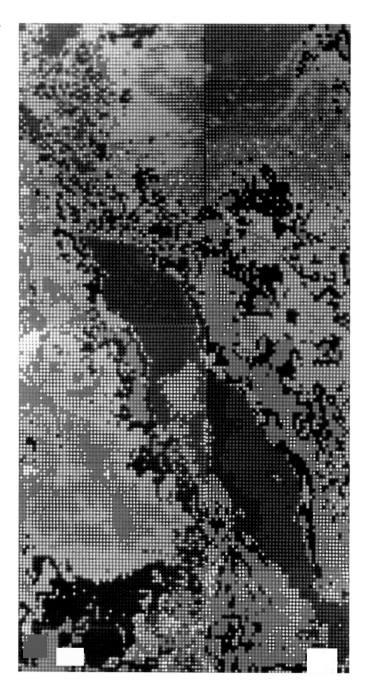

The processing is parallel in the sense that all the squares are examined and compared with the stored patterns at once. However, it is a relatively simple form of parallel processing. The array processor does not actually do anything that a suitably programmed general-purpose computer cannot do.

Networks have been around since the early 1960s. Paul Weston's program Cylinders (circa 1965) at the University of Illinois simulated an organization similar to, and in many ways more sophisticated than, the rings of today. Oliver Selfridge's Pandemonium, developed at the Massachusetts Institute of Technology and described at a British Physical Laboratory Symposium in 1959, was an expert system. And probably the earliest array processors were a range of devices called Perceptrons, built by Frank Rosenblatt at Cornell University throughout the 1960s.

The novelty of the current generation of computers is more technical than theoretical, although the original ideas have been greatly refined over the years. Using microelectronics it is possible (and practical) to connect many computing elements together in any of the ways we have outlined.

The number of machines in a system may be very large. For example, there are rings or nets that contain 60 or more computers. An expert system made up in the way we describe could easily have 100 experts. Some array processors work with a two-dimensional array of 12 x 15 elements, and even larger devices have been constructed, such as Clip 4 at Imperial College, London.

Conflict

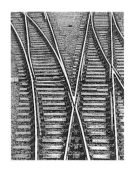

The great divide between simple forms of parallel processing – those that do not enable the computer to think in any but a logical, deductive way – and more complex arrangements – that may open up the possibility of other thought patterns – comes at the point where conflict enters the picture.

What do we mean by conflict? Basically, that two or more time sequences of computation, which may have been proceeding in parallel, interact. Instead of remaining parallel and (by the definition of parallel) separate, they converge in a head-on collision from which there is no logical-deductive retreat.

Let us look in some detail at a program, the game of Life, that illustrates some of the differences between serial and parallel operation and shows how conflict might occur. John Conway, a British mathematician with an interest in patterns and the nature of order, was its inventor.

The game of Life takes place on a checkerboard (no different, you will note, from an array) on which each square can be 'on' or 'off', black or white. The game starts with the player designating a number of squares as on (shown as black in the diagrams). It then proceeds in time phases (moves). In each phase, every square on the board is checked, and some are altered, according to the state of neighbouring cells in the previous phase. A square is switched on if, and only if, exactly three of its immediate neighbouring squares (including diagonal squares) were on in the previous phase. Squares already on continue to 'live' if two or three neighbouring cells were on. If none, one, or four or more neighbouring cells were on, a square 'dies' and is switched off.

The drawings below show the start of a game, the opening configuration (chosen by the player) and the next three phases. You will see that a pattern emerges from the apparently random opening arrangement. (You may like to follow the development of the pattern, by working out the next two phases).

The start of a Life game. Can you fill in stages 5 and 6, abiding by the rules given above?

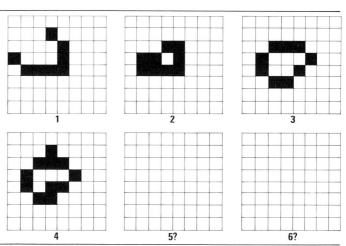

1 2 3

4 5? 6?

How might the game of Life be programmed on a computer? The computing it requires could be handled (at least from a functional viewpoint) by three alternative types of system corresponding to some of the systems we have explored already.

First, it could be handled by a network of microprocessors working in parallel, but in a co-ordinated fashion. Each microprocessor might take one square, then, at a designated instant all the microprocessors would determine the state of their square in the next phase, and all the squares would switch to the next phase.

Alternatively, it could be handled by an array processor, using an array of the same size as the checkerboard. The array processor would carry out all the testing and switching involved in one phase in parallel.

Or it could be handled on a serial computer, but not simply by telling it to look at each square in turn and change its state if necessary. Whatever the order in which the squares were looked at, the results of earlier moves would affect later moves and an incorrect pattern would emerge, and so the serial computer would have to simulate the parallel processing done by the other two types of set-up. This could be done by telling it to set up a storage area consisting of locations in one-to-one correspondence with the squares of the checkerboard. Then it would examine each square on the board in turn and indicate the square's state in the next phase of the game, not by changing it on the board, but by recording the data in the store. When it had examined all the squares, it could clear the checkerboard, and copy all the data in the storage area onto the board again.

One would hardly use a real network of computers in the way just described, but the game of Life illustrates three ways in which parallel processing can be carried out. In none of these three methods is there any apparent conflict: the processing tasks are clearly separated, and as long as they are well synchronized there would seem to be no problem. However, it is easy to demonstrate how a simple conflict might occur. What if two microprocessors both examined the same set of squares using slightly different criteria to decide whether they should be on or off? One of them might employ a variation on our rules that says cells should switched on if they have either three or four 'on' neighbours. The processors would clearly disagree over some squares, one wishing to have them on, and the other to turn them off. Result: a conflict that the machines themselves could not, apparently, solve.

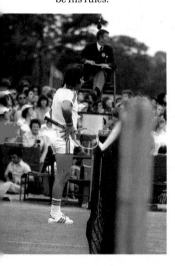

My rules don't seem to be his rules.

Patterns and concepts

The game of Life also illustrates another important idea, that of patterns, which in turn leads to the idea of concept formation. Take a look at the drawings opposite which show successive phases in a real game. You will probably find it difficult to take in every detail of the play, but clustering the black squares together in your mind, and focusing on these dominant features, you make some sense of the state of play very quickly. And you interpret each cluster as being continuous from one picture to the next, even though the clusters are made up of different squares. This has parallels with theories of how concepts are built up in the human mind, a question we shall explore later. You recognize ways in which the patterns extend and develop, but you can also identify specific patterns that

A sequence of moves from a real Life game; how many distinct patterns can you identify? What is the sense or the dimension that enables us to recognize consistency, development, change, interaction, conflict and resolution?

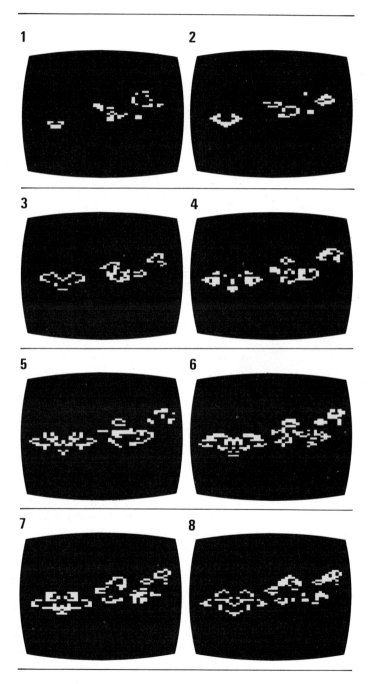

re-occur. They may occur at precisely the same location on the checkerboard, or they may migrate around the board, and a number of different sequences may lead to the production of the same pattern.

The concept of self-reproduction – of patterns which reproduce themselves – was first formalized around 1955 by the great cybernetic theorist John von Neumann in the United States. He used a number of models, some like Conway's model, and some quite different. The concept was later explored by, among others, American theorists Arthur Burkes and Edgar Codd. In the 1960s Lars Loefgren in Sweden extended von Neumann's work, to demonstrate the possibility of evolutionary organizations. These are patterns that not only reproduce themselves, but also produce a number (an arbitrarily large number) of new types of pattern, that are in turn self-reproducing.

With the identification of groups of squares, which can be seen as patterns-concepts that we distinguish from other patterns-concepts on the checkerboard, we encounter the prospect of a new type of conflict. Just as our hypothetical rival microprocessors interacted to produce conflict over particular squares, so we find whole patterns colliding. In this two-dimensional universe, it is common for patterns to interact destructively; by recognizing the integrity of different patterns, we also recognize conflict when they collide.

There is a useful analogy between conflicting patterns developing on the checkerboard and conflicting programs running in the same computer. Some programming languages introduce the concept of a 'virtual computer'. This means that the programmer can designate part of the computer's processing and storage capacity as a separate entity, on which a program and the data needed by it can be stored and run. The virtual computer does not simply take over a geographical or chronological chunk of the computer's capacity. It changes in both location and content as the program is being run, just as the patterns on the Life game board change while the program is running. A virtual computer is no more than a concept; it has no specific existence in hardware terms. But our identification of it as a concept enables us to recognize its continuing existence in spite of its changing content and location.

By setting up several virtual computers within the same real computer, the programmer can run more than one program at once on the same microprocessor, just as more than one pattern at a time develops on the checkerboard. Just as patterns can conflict on the checkerboard, conflict between virtual computers can occur. This is serious because it may cause one program to interfere with the accuracy of another's processing operations.

To extend the analogy, it is perfectly reasonable to think of the patterns on the checkerboard as being computers themselves. At each phase the patterns display input (the pattern of the previous phase, and the rules of the game), carry out processing, and display output (the new pattern). This interpretation is not far-fetched, provided we keep in mind the fact that our simple example was chosen for the sake of clarity rather than utility. In fact, the data input and the pattern's reaction to it quite closely resemble the events that occur when a pattern (for example, a script character displayed on retina of a photoelectric device) is input to an array processor.

It is therefore reasonable to ask whether any method of resolving conflicts between patterns on a checkerboard might be applicable to virtual computers, and to other types of conflict. If so, what would such conflict resolution entail? Apart from an identification of the patterns as autonomous units, essential to the concept of conflict, it would demand two major features: first, some way for the patterns to know that they are likely to interact destructively, even though they are not yet touching; and second, some room for bargaining. That is, the patterns must have the opportunity to alter the rules of the checkerboard universe, for example by redefining the concept of 'neighbouring cells' or by changing the spatial characteristics of the checker-board. Conflict resolution would be possible if such bargaining took place, and if there were at least one mutually satisfactory modification.

Patterns and virtual computers are not the only entities that might conflict. At the moment microprocessors and array processors are used almost exclusively in conflict-free ways. However, there are many areas in which a broader conception of computing and computers might lead to uses that bring compu-ter components into conflict. Using computers in such ways makes it essential to develop methods for resolving conflict.

Thought patterns and consciousness

One way of considering the human mind is to say that it works in a way that opens up the possibility both of conflict and conflict resolution.

Many early researchers in artificial intelligence (notably Warren McCulloch of the Massachusetts Institute of Technology, Ross Ashby, Alan Newell, Herbert Simon and Edward Feigen-baum) were anxious to model computing systems on what is known of the workings of the human brain in the hope that such systems would exhibit intelligent behaviour. Sadly, our know-ledge of the human brain and its workings is far from complete and these early experiments did much to teach us that the neuron networks of the brain are not as simple as we once believed they might be.

This approach to simulating human brain activity was largely superseded by attempts to model behaviour instead. In other words, artificial intelligence systems attempted to reproduce the results of human thought processes without necessarily (perhaps without ever) using the brain's methods of achieving them. The original researchers tried to work forwards, from the thought processes to their result in the form of intelligent behaviour. Their successors tried to work backwards from intelligent behaviour to the processes that produce it.

Today the tide is turning, and both kinds of approach are used to complement each other. This became evident in the latest NATO artificial intelligence symposium, held in Lyon (France) in 1981.

As a result of these historical developments, artificial intelligence applies many of the concepts we use in talking about human thought without necessarily building up to them in the same way as the human brain. Concept formation is one such concept. Another is the idea of consciousness.

What is consciousness? You will probably agree that it is being aware of what you are thinking or doing. You look at what you are thinking from another dimension, from an external perspective, almost as you look at a film. And because you know what you think or do, as well as thinking and doing, you are able to adapt your thinking and doing, to learn from experience.

Marvin Minsky, one of the most celebrated specialists in

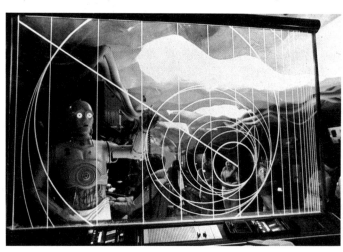

Dimensions within dimensions, from the film The Empire Strikes Back. *Much science fantasy is scientifically spurious but it demonstrates the human brain's staggering capacity for association and extrapolation. Aided by computers, where will our creativity lead us?*

The start of a Bach fugue in which the melodies interweave and interact. A practised player of fugues indulges in parallel as well as interactive processing.

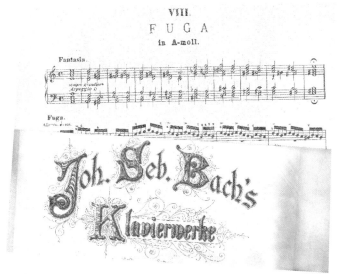

Hand with reflecting globe, an engraving by M.C. Escher. We all hold models of ourselves inside our heads and feel distressed and confused when they do not match up.

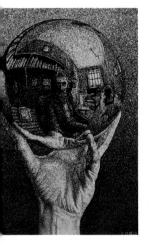

artificial intelligence, put it in computer terms by saying that consciousness is the ability of a system to hold a model, or even several models, of itself and its behaviour.

We have encountered this idea before, in two different guises. First, take the serial computer carrying out the game of Life. It sets up, you recall, a separate storage area which it uses as a model of the checkerboard. The storage area may seem a facile concept but in fact it provides a whole new dimension to the computer's processing power. It could be thought of as a new space dimension, as a checkerboard parallel to, but not intersecting, the original board. It could be thought of as a time dimension, enabling the processor to carry out a series of moves in the one instant of the switch from one game phase to the next. Or again, it could be seen as analogous with consciousness. Think about it.

We came across the same idea when discussing conflict resolution. What do we need in order to resolve the conflict between two interacting patterns? A model of the two patterns and their behaviour, an external perspective on their interaction.

The model need not be within a separate machine. Our brains do not need a separate extension to be conscious of their own workings. Similarly, a computer can manage to hold (in a virtual computer) a model of a different dimension of its own processing activities. It seems clear, too, that areas of our brain adopt distinct personalities, rather like the distinct virtual computers within a single computer or the distinct patterns on the checkerboard. We resolve conflict by mediating between these distinct personalities.

This notion was put forward by the British neurophysiologist Grey Walter (whom we meet again) in the middle 1950s, and investigated later by measuring electrical activity in the brains of people with surgically implanted electrodes. It seems that when the brain is working, groups of neurons, each with their own coherent activity patterns, interact with each other. When the electrical activity of different areas of the brain is measured, there are significant variations between them, but these variations disappear just before an action takes place or a problem is solved. The decrease in variation can be monitored by computer, and used to enable the computer to react more rapidly than a human being in critical circumstances — for example when a bomber pilot recognizes his target.

A common model of thought processes, dialectical reasoning, shows some interesting parallels with this phenomenon. The German philosopher Hegel brought dialectics, a Greek mode of debate, into philosophy as a model of reasoning. Basically, dialectic interprets reasoning as the reaching of a synthesis between an original idea, the thesis, and an opposing idea, the antithesis. The thesis is the original proposal, and the antithesis is a statement which apparently contradicts it. There is conflict as long as thesis and antithesis try to coexist in the same world of thought. Synthesis resolves the conflict. The part of our mind that synthesizes must be aware of the content of both thesis and antithesis; it resolves a conflict between two personalities in the brain, one upholding the thesis and the other the antithesis.

A fluorescing microscope picture of living computer fabric: a network of neurons.

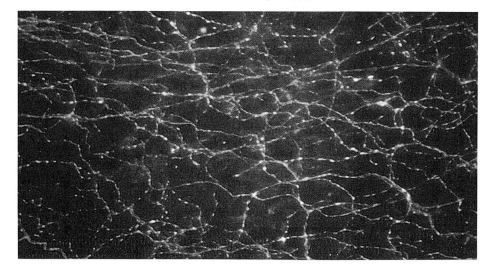

Many theorists would agree that many of our thought processes can be described in this way, although this means taking the dialectical model somewhat further than many orthodox philosophers would wish. Unfortunately such a model does not clarify the question of how we actually reach synthesis. Is it always by logical deduction? One could argue that juxtaposing an improbable thesis and antithesis sometimes leads to creative synthesis. As an exercise in dialectical reasoning we might bring together such diametrically opposed models of creative thought processes as Edward de Bono's 'lateral thinking' and Arthur Koestler's 'association of ideas', one the thesis and the other the antithesis. And we might find that creativity is less far removed from logical thought than we sometimes suppose. If this is the case, it might one day be possible to make computers behave in ways that appear to be, or indeed are, creative.

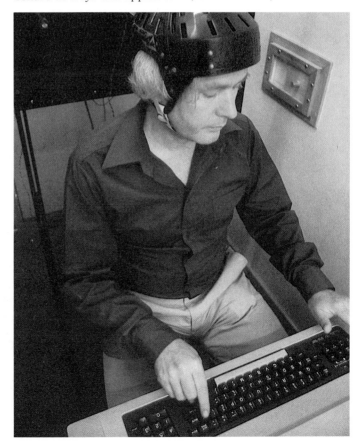

Which part of the brain does what, and when? The electrodes inside this helmet register activity in the cortex or outer rind of the brain and display it on the light board behind. Visual, verbal and spatial tasks trigger off activity in corresponding parts of the cortex.

Chapter 4 POPULATIONS OF COMPUTERS

What is a memorable concept? We mean by this a concept that remains in long-term memory, in contrast to a telephone number, remembered for the time it takes to dial it and then forgotten. A concept is an abstract or general idea that we use to organize our thoughts and experiences, in much the same way that we used the patterns on the checkerboard on page 65 to organize our perception of what was happening.

But there are other aspects of a concept that are worth stressing. First, a concept is possessed by an individual. The words we use to designate concepts are common to many individuals but the content of each person's concept is unique. Our concept of a factory will not be the same as your concept of a factory, though our concepts have enough in common to make it possible for us to discuss factories without confusion.

Second, most of our concepts are in flux. We develop and adapt them as we go along. We try to form them into a reasonably ordered hierarchy of ideas and experiences, and in general we adopt a pragmatic attitude to overlaps.

Third, we build elaborate concepts out of simple concepts, although not necessarily by the same route. 'Factory' to you might primarily mean 'building', 'product', 'process' and 'manager', while to us it might conjure up 'product', 'assembly line', 'manager' and 'building'. We both arrive at the same concept by a different route, and use slightly different building blocks. In a comparable way, there are many routes that lead to the same pattern in the Life game. Each component of a concept is also a concept, in turn built up of many components that are also concepts, and so on.

Present-day computers do not possess anything like the richness of the human conceptual system. Nevertheless by applying what we know of the process of concept formation and

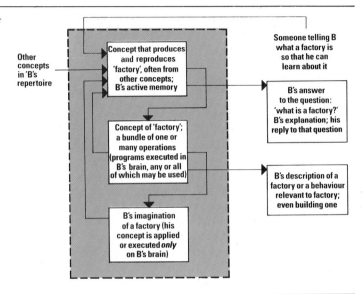

One person's concept of 'factory'. A concept is a more or less coherent collection (the shaded area) of many other personalized and multi-faceted concepts.

Other concepts in 'B's repertoire

Concept that produces and reproduces 'factory', often from other concepts; B's active memory

Concept of 'factory'; a bundle of one or many operations (programs executed in B's brain, any or all of which may be used)

B's imagination of a factory (his concept is applied or executed *only* on B's brain)

Someone telling B what a factory is so that he can learn about it

B's answer to the question: 'what is a factory?' B's explanation; his reply to that question

B's description of a factory or a behaviour relevant to factory; even building one

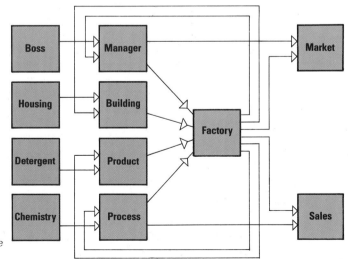

One person's mesh of concepts, including the concept 'factory'. The boxes in this diagram represent the contents of the shaded area in the diagram above.

Boss

Manager

Market

Housing

Building

Factory

Detergent

Product

Chemistry

Process

Sales

adaptation to techniques of computer programming it should be possible to produce computers which think, in the sense of being able to resolve conflict. Much of human thinking involves the resolution of conflict – knowing one thing and feeling another, deciding on priorities, choosing between alternatives.

Concepts, in both humans and computers, are a fertile source of conflict; we assume we are talking about the same thing, but in fact we are applying the same label to concepts with somewhat different contents. However, if we exchange information about the contents of our concepts we have a tool for resolving the incompatibilities between us. Similarly, if a computer has a model of its concepts, it too has a tool for resolving the incompatibilities between them and making them mesh together. Conflict resolution in a computer may be primitive compared to the amazingly flexible and complex conflict resolution that goes on in the human brain but it is nonetheless real.

Our purpose in this chapter is to show that independent computers are capable of creating and to some extent resolving conflict when they are arranged so that they interact with each other. We call an arrangement of computers that does this an 'independent population of computers'. The word independent is important here. For what distinguishes a population of computers from the net and ring structures described earlier is the absence of a common controller. In a conventional net or ring the controller ensures that conflict between the different processors in the network does not occur. If there is no controller, and processing operations are not synchronized and running in parallel, the way is open for conflict. The way is also open for individual members of the population to interact in ways which the presence of a controller would not permit. A very famous early experiment by the British neurophysiologist Grey Walter explored exactly this possibility.

Grey Walter worked at the Burden Neurological Institute near Bristol and he had a penchant for electromechanical gadgetry. In the early 1950s he built a number of small battery-powered robots called 'tortoises'. Each of them contained a simple but powerful computing system, basically analog in structure. They were able to move freely round the floor, and were able to sense light signals and solid objects as they did so. When their batteries ran low they would head towards a recharging station, to which they were attracted by a light. They were quite independent of one another – their computing circuitry was not physically linked in any way – but they were capable of interacting. Although programmed to avoid solid objects, they occasionally bumped into one another. Their light

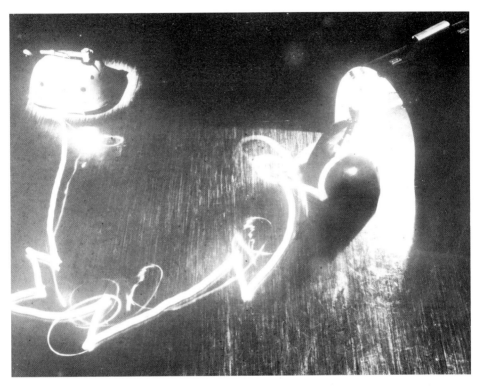

A time-lapse photograph of one of Grey Walter's tortoises making tracks towards the recharging station.

sensors also occasionally confused the light of the recharging station with the flashing lights on their own heads which indicated that their batteries were running low. Within the frame of reference of their system collisions and confusions counted as examples of conflict.

It was particularly interesting to see what happened when two tortoises collided and were unable to escape from the situation. Typically a third tortoise would move in and by its presence break the deadlock. In general the behaviour of the tortoises was co-operative, primitive though it may have been by human standards, and showed a richness difficult to reconcile with the simplicity of their structure.

For the possibilities it opens up of co-operation, if for no other reason in this uncertain world, it would be wise to explore the idea of populations of computers.

Co-operative systems of this kind constitute a sub-class of what Heinz von Foerster of the Biological Computer Laboratory, University of Illinois, has called 'self-organizing systems'. Though often loosely used to refer to systems that are adaptive, the term self-organizing accords in its strictest sense with an independent reinvention of von Foerster's definition by John Nicolis of the University of Patras, Greece: 'If a system is self-organizing, then the rate of change of a suitable measure of its organization is positive'. For our purposes a positive rate of change of 'a suitable measure of organization' can be taken as meaning the active co-operation through interaction of the individuals constituting a computer population. Thus, Grey Walter's tortoises interacted co-operatively.

However, if any population continues to organize itself there comes a point when it is fully organized. It will then cease to be self-organizing. If it is to continue to be self-organizing there must be the possibility of growth. In effect the population must be capable of generating or finding new independent members that can become part of it and organize themselves with it. To compensate for the increasing dependency through co-operative interaction of its individual members the population as a whole must create or capture new members. Usually these two conditions – dependency and annexation – go on together in balance.

A very primitive self-organizing system: the single-celled amoeba. The organelles and other components of single cells are as much a co-operative population as the millions of cells in the human body.

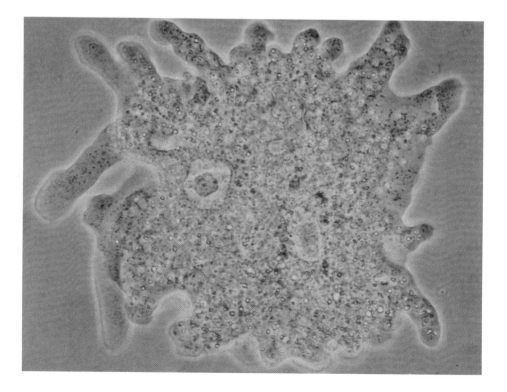

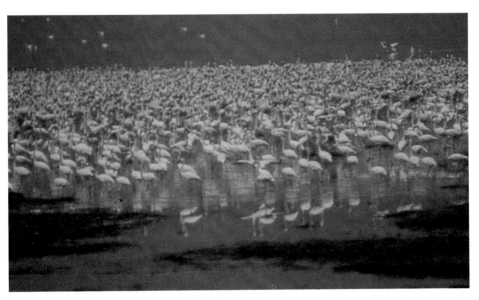

Every animal population treads a fine line between dependency on its habitat and the ability to adapt by maintaining and introducing genetic variety.

For computers to co-operate fruitfully in order to solve a problem, or in order to maintain certain conditions in a changing world, they need to bring independent and different perspectives to the task. In essence, they will have to have different programs and these will inevitably conflict with each other. But if the conflict can be resolved the problem stands a chance of being solved too.

This idea is central to the concept of a population of computers. A population of computers would be self-organizing in a way that increased both the amount of conflict and the amount of conflict resolution. And to continue to be self-organizing the population would have to generate or capture additional units equipped with different, conflict-promoting programs. In principle the fecundity of a population of computers would be unlimited; in practice it would be limited by the number of capturable machines and programs available.

Grey Walter's population of tortoises clearly did not embody all the requirements of a self-organizing system – there were no capturable tortoises – but the population we are about to describe does embody them, in a very simple way.

A Colloquy of Mobiles

In 1968 Jasia Reichardt, then Director of the Institute of Contemporary Arts in London, asked Gordon Pask to build an exhibit for an exhibition. The title of the exhibition was Cybernetic Serendipity and it included robots, Peter Zenovief's computer-generated music, Herbert Brun's computer graphics, and many other cybernetic displays. Jasia asked for something that would illustrate tangibly Pask's ideas (thought very strange at the time) about co-operative action and self-organization. If possible, it should have some aesthetic merit. The result was an exhibit called A Colloquy of Mobiles. This represented an ecological, or perhaps an ethological, fantasy.

The Colloquy covered a floor area of 15 x 12 feet (5 x 4 metres) and consisted of five powered mobiles suspended from powered beams 11 feet (3.75 metres) above the ground. It was therefore big enough for people to walk into and interact with. It was intended for operation in the dark or under fairly dim lighting conditions.

Although all the mobiles were physically identical, they interacted in a way which suggested that two were male and three were female. The object of their programs was to mate with a mobile of the opposite sex, and their interaction consisted primarily of competing for the mate of their choice. In the restricted territory allowed by the suspension beams, this frequently led to conflict.

All the mobiles were equipped with several photoelectric cells which could emit a light beam, modulated by a dimmer. They also had vertically scanning light reflectors and could rotate horizontally on their centre axes. The suspension beams, which determined the positions of the mobiles' centres, could also be moved. To effect movement, the mobiles had to expend power – a metaphor, if you like, for a human male or female spending money in search of a mate.

The mobiles contained what would nowadays be called microprocessors, programmed in different ways to achieve the same goal. They could accept programs from the micro-processors in any other mobile, but only if the two mobiles had interacted in a predefined way.

Pask also built in a primitive method of expanding the population as organization (mating, in this case) took place. It would have been too expensive to generate fresh mobiles as the result of male-female intercourse, so one female always stayed inactive unless the interaction between the others lapsed, at which point 'she' became active.

The mobiles did indeed exhibit a form of societal interplay. They behaved as something more than an arbitrary collection of robots; from the way they interacted it appeared that they shared information and thus formed a corporate organization, a self-organizing society. The exhibition ran for four months, though the mobiles, poor things, needed repairing every few days.

Gordon Pask,
Colloquy of Mobiles,
1968.

In order to remain a self-organizing system the mobiles had to steer a middle course between two extremes: no conflict resolution, in which case the system would fail to organize at all; and total organization, total sharing of information, in which case the individual character of the machines would be destroyed. The introduction of the stand-by mobile and of the human element was a safeguard against total organization.

Let us restate this scenario from a slightly different perspective. Conflict cannot be resolved except by communication, by some sharing of concepts, whether that sharing takes place between people, between processors, or between people and processors. But sharing must not be carried to the point where all distinction between the sharers is lost. That would be coalescence, not communication.

It should be possible to share concepts with other people in such a way that the shared part can be represented as a process in a population of machines. The interaction between human communicators and machines would then be conversational in character.

This can be exemplified by looking at the way in which visitors to Cybernetic Serendipity interacted with the Colloquy of Mobiles. Here are some of the answers people gave when asked about their reactions to the mobiles: 'Played with them', 'Liked (or disliked) one or other of them', 'Danced with them', 'Formed coalitions with them, and with other participants', 'Learned their private language, and communicated in it' by blocking off the light beams emitted by the mobiles' photoelectric cells.

Although the mobiles' language was a simple one, it enabled interaction to take place. Some visitors stayed in the mobiles' enclosure for hours on end. Did they really communicate with the mobiles, or the mobiles with them? Did they interact with, or merely act upon, the mobiles? Did they impose personalities, or project their own personalities, on them? Did they use them to resolve their own inner conflicts?

The answers to these questions are not obvious. Human interaction with the mobiles certainly modified interaction between the mobiles, and in that sense the humans contributed to the self-organizing society in which the mobiles were the central figures.

But what would have happened if those taking part had lacked the information contained in the mobiles' processors? Without that information the behaviour of the mobiles would not have been predictable. The mobiles would not have acted like pawns moving round a chess board representing the externalized thought processes of the humans present. Instead they would have stubbornly stuck to 'ideas' of their own about how they wished to move, and the unpredictability of their responses might have modified the thought processes of their human audience.

This possibility raises several questions of a more general nature. Can we hold a real conversation with a computer if it has been programmed to ask and answer questions in ways that we cannot predict? Would we merely be talking to the ghost of the programmer, or to ourselves? If neither, we would surely be talking to the computer itself. We would undoubtedly find our thoughts influenced by our interaction with the computer. At that moment we would become micro men.

Broadening the scope of computation

The concern with conflict-free operations that prevails throughout most of the computer industry today is entirely understandable. Such operations are appropriate when the object of calculation is to yield logically true or false results, or where industrial processes have to be kept within strictly controlled limits. Control necessarily relies on computation based on the factually true and false. Even statistical predictions of the kind required by design engineers or weather forecasters, in which true and false are probables rather than absolutes, are founded on conflict-free operations.

Just as the first computers were mostly dedicated to the production of mathematical tables, so present-day computers are primarily conceived of as devices that manipulate numbers and symbols and give results that are logically or factually true. Programs are written to satisfy criteria of correctness; they terminate at a fixed point, and may then be repeated using fresh values of data. A process control program, for instance, regularly re-tests the process being carried out; it then uses the results of the tests to update the process variables.

There is nothing wrong with this attitude towards computation. It does, however, lead to an unnecessarily blinkered view of what computation is. It encourages a tendency to regard computer applications that do not rely on true-false criteria as somehow suspect, with the result that disappointingly little effort is channelled into less conventional areas.

There are many areas in which conflict-resolving computation could be extremely useful. For example, it is often necessary to give and obey commands; ask and answer questions; reason by analogy; obtain statements of agreement; forecast future possibilities rather than assign probability values to already chosen scenarios; formulate problems rather than solve problems already formulated. All of these activities could be carried out by

Opposite:
'A new symbolical head and phrenological chart with the name and definition of each organ'. Natural philosophers of the past thought of the brain as containing many distinct personalities. The author of this nineteenth century engraving postulated organs of 'amativeness', 'conjugality', 'parental love', 'sublimity', 'ideality', 'tune', 'destructiveness', and many more.

computers, but attempts to carry them out in conflict-free systems will be at best approximations and sometimes unproductive or even misleading.

We glibly talk of computers asking or answering questions, of issuing commands. We do not really believe that a conventional computer can ask or answer questions or give commands in the same way that a human being can. The computer is only engaging in a simple logical-deductive process which superficially resembles answering, questioning, and commanding. What about computer systems embodying forms of thought based on conflict resolution? Their answers, questions, and commands would not be the outcome of logical deduction.

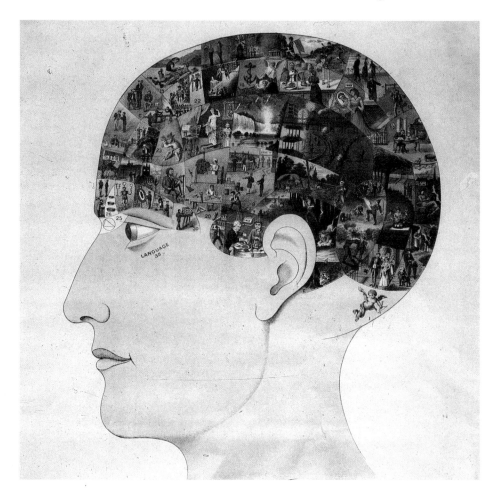

To press the point home, let us consider the following statement: 'Smith told Jones to stand on the box when the bell rang; the bell rang and Jones stood on the box'. Smith may or may not have told Jones to stand on the box, and Jones may or may not have obeyed – we do not know whether either piece of information is true or false. But, true or false, we know that the events the statement purports to describe are undoubtedly in the past. In itself the statement is not a command or a display of obedience, although it certainly contains both ideas. In fact, it bears the same tangential relationship to command and obedience as a conventionally programmed computer does to the content of its program. The computer may be programmed to print a selected piece of text with an exclamation mark or a question mark after it, but it is not commanding or questioning us. It is merely relaying the programmer's command or question after the event.

What if the programmer were unable to predict the content of the computer's response? Would the command or question truly be that of the computer? It would certainly not be the programmer's. As more complex and many-levelled artificial intelligence programs are developed we will find that what we comfortably assumed to be purely metaphorical commands, questions and answers come to resemble real commands, questions and answers. Attempts to produce machines that think mean that the differences between people and machines have to be re-evaluated. Do computers think in significantly different ways from humans, and is it desirable that they should? Thought is not necessarily or uniquely a property of biological fabric. To many workers in the field of artificial intelligence, thought is an activity that can reasonably be assumed to go on in a variety of natural and constructed systems. Some systems are biological, as our brain is; some are not biological, but microelectronic. Some of this thought is conventional computation, but some of it is not. Much that is not conventional computation cannot be accommodated, by principle of design, in any one standard computer, but it could be accommodated in a population of computers.

Chapter **5 LANGUAGE & KNOWLEDGE**

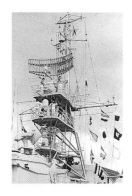

Flags and radar aboard a modern frigate. Flags are still used to send signals from ship to ship though systems vary from navy to navy.

Making a computer 'think' is all very well. But what is the computer to think about? If computers are to help us solve real problems, they must have some knowledge of the real world. We shall look at knowledge in the form of language and ponder how it can be used as a basis for making computers think.

A language is a way of representing the concepts that make up a body of knowledge. It does not have to contain words. Gestures used in a consistent way form the basis of sign languages (like deaf, dumb and mime languages). Other symbols – numbers, chess pieces, religious totems – can also be used consistently to form the basis of a language

You may feel that this definition of language is close to your own but not identical. That is not surprising. There are many differences between what individuals and groups of individuals mean by a given word. However, what we mean by 'language' and what you mean by 'language' are sufficiently similar for us to agree upon the use of the word.

There is a difficulty, however. We have defined our concept of language in words, but words themselves stand for concepts to which we attach slightly different meanings. The concepts you label 'concept', 'knowledge' and even 'word' will not be identical to concepts we label 'concepts', 'knowledge' or 'word'. And the more precisely we try to use such labels the more obvious our differences become. Escaping from this trap and finding a set of concept labels – a language – which has the same meaning to everyone has been the aim of philosophers for centuries.

Public knowledge

The view of many classical philosophers, a view derived from Plato, was that for every concept there is an ideal definition, a definition which captures its essence. There is an ideal chair, even an ideal idea. The individual chairs and ideas from which we build up our definitions of chair and idea all differ to some extent from the ideal. But in a public language, one used by many people, the ideals are the essences of the concepts we all share. Thus, there is a right way to use the word chair or idea. There is a right word to describe every individual object.

Imagine two people looking at the same pot of paint. One says it is red and the other says it is orange. Neither is lying; they just differ over where to divide the spectrum into red and orange. According to the classical view of language, one of them is wrong. According to our view, neither is wrong.

The classical view assumes that words are just as real and definite as objects like factories and actions like building factories. Words of course do refer to concrete objects and specific happenings, but this does not make the words themselves concrete or specific.

Coherency and truth

The fact that some people still hold the classical view of language helps to account for their confusion when they try to decide if what comes out of a computer is the truth. The table of attitudes on page 52 shows that 30 per cent of those interviewed believed that 'computers can produce results that are more accurate than the information they are given'. Even allowing for the tendency we all have to trust words in print or on a video screen, this is a remarkable figure. Somewhere along the line truth and consistency have been confused.

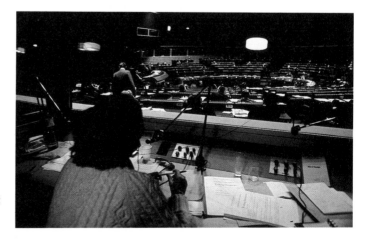

Huge bureaucracies such as the EEC and United Nations would crumble overnight were it not for teams of translators making consistent and coherent links between different languages.

If a language is to function at all it must operate in a consistent and coherent way. By and large words must mean the same thing each time they are used, so that they can be used to build up larger meanings such as sentences and arguments. In a coherent system the parts do not contradict the whole.

A scientific hypothesis works in the same way. It forms a logical framework into which evidence is fitted. The hypothesis need not be true; it is useful as long as the system based on it is not exposed as contrary, since this would destroy its coherence. One can take a similar view of religious beliefs; they work as long as they are self-consistent. One reason for the resilience of religions and entrenched schools of scientific thought is that they are coherent, though their coherence is more social than intellectual. Evidence contrary to the prevailing system is rejected or distorted into favourable evidence. Only an insurmountable volume of inconsistent material will destroy the system.

To further demonstrate the distinction between truth and coherence, take the fictional world of *Lord of the Rings*. We do not mistake it for the real world but it is so coherent and complete that we can sustain belief in it through hundreds of pages. Had Tolkien made a small mistake, and described a journey incompatible at some point with the topography of his created world, we would probably overlook the contrary evidence. However, had he introduced a new topography with every chapter we would be very confused indeed, with no system into which to fit our knowledge of his fictional world.

Knowledge can be defined as a structured body of concepts which can be expressed in a public or private language; the concepts must be common and shared and form a coherent system but they need not be true. Knowledge, to us, includes not only verified concepts, but also hypotheses, beliefs and out-and-out fictions. (If you take issue with this use of knowledge please substitute a word you prefer throughout the rest of this book.)

Since a computer operates in a logical way the language in which it is programmed must be logically consistent. That does not mean that the concepts expressed by the language have to be true. To the computer that is irrelevant. The computer usually does not know what the concepts consist of, only that the symbols are used consistently and make up a coherent system. The result of the computer's processing will obey the rules of this logical system, but be no more true than the system itself. What the computer does is manipulate symbols, and these symbols may stand for facts or fictions. In this sense the computer is always making models of systems, not reproducing them.

It is vital to bear this distinction in mind when thinking about computer simulations. A simulation is a model specifically intended to represent truth in a particular sphere, whether in finance, meteorology or astrophysics. Confusion sometimes occurs when, for example, managers have direct access to models of economic or stocktaking processes. They may say things such as 'The simulation told me to do such and such' or 'The model was to blame', forgetting that they are dealing only with a model, whose results they themselves must test and validate in the real world.

Full and empty symbols

Words like 'factory' or 'bicycle' represent different, though analogous, concepts to different people. Are all concepts as variable in their content? Are there some concepts that are ideal, some concepts that have the same label and the same content for everybody?

This too is a central question in philosophy; for if we can be certain that we are talking about the same thing, we can get down in earnest to finding out whether what we are talking about is true. However, the search for ideal concepts has proved difficult. It is relatively easy to construct a coherent system, a formal logic like algebra, in which we manipulate empty symbools such as a, b and c according to a consistent set of rules. Once we assign meanings to a, b and c it is not so easy to decide whether our logical model is a true representation of events in a real world. In other words, there is no problem in manipulating empty symbols. The problem arises when we try to manipulate 'full' symbols or symbols with fixed meanings that are, in some specific context, true as well as consistent.

A concept like 4 is rather different; 4 is not an empty symbol like x in algebra. It has a definite meaning and it seems highly likely that this meaning is the same for all of us. Number systems do represent a real world for which we can attempt to create a true language.

Formal and natural language

The language of whole numbers is a formal language; the symbols and the way in which they can be manipulated are fully defined. Any language that specifies all the ways in which the letters A to Z, and a selection of signs like ,!?;: can be manipulated is also a formal language. Computer languages are like this. The question of truth does not enter into their construction; they consist of empty symbols. Truth and falsehood only come into the picture when we assign meanings to the symbols, and attempt to compare the working of our language model with events in the real world.

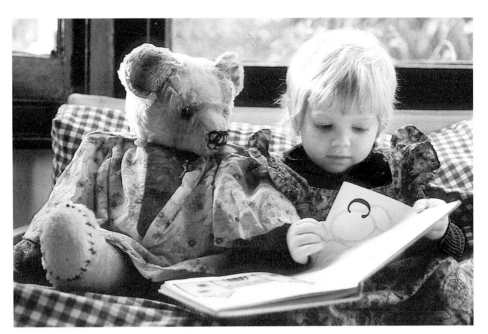

Truth and fiction are all one to bears and little girls. But the world this little girl has created for herself has a logic of its own, as any intruding adult will quickly discover.

It is, for example, perfectly possible to construct a logical language in which we can make such statements as '4 - 2 = 8' and 'black is white'. The rules allow such statements provided they do not contradict the logic of the system. Both statements only become untrue when we give meanings to the symbols and find that the perfectly logical statements we have created do not reflect the truth of the real world. In the same way, they become true only when the meanings we assign to them result in the statements that *do* reflect truth in the real world. Give the symbol 4 the usual meaning of 10 and give the symbol 'black' the usual meaning of 'snow', let everything else mean what it normally means, and both statements are correct.

All statements in computer language are converted into binary code for the computer to manipulate. One instruction in a high-level language such as PASCAL or BASIC may convert to a long string of binary ones and zeros in machine code. But however complicated it is, the resulting machine code is unchanging. If the instruction ADD in BASIC is converted into 001000001 in machine code on a specific computer, then it will always be converted to 001000001 and never to 001000011. ADD is a fully defined symbol since it always produces that particular machine code, which will always cause the computer to carry out the same operation(s).

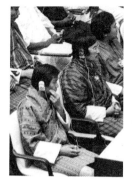

The same is true of data; these also have to be converted into binary ones and zeros before the computer can manipulate them. It does not matter that a particular code stands for 'truth', 'beauty', or some other concept which it might take volumes to define. To the computer that code is fully defined, part of its formal language. We could store on a computer all the letters that make up this book in sequence and converted into binary. In this form the computer could manipulate the contents of the book because the codes are part of its formal language and it has fully defined rules for manipulating them. To human readers, however, the letters carry a message that is much less well defined. But that is of no consequence to the computer; it does not have to understand our concepts in order to manipulate the symbols that represent them.

In this very special sense languages like French, English or Italian can be treated as formal languages. When we come to consider the meanings that such natural languages convey, however, they are far from formal. It is by no means easy even to formalize the rules of grammar to produce an exhaustive and unambiguous set of rules about how words may be combined.

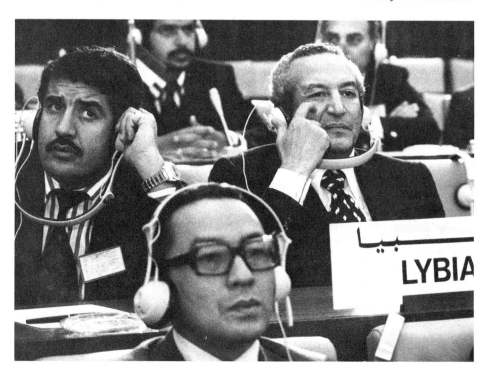

Language to computer

There is nothing inherently wrong with models. Architectural models and the aircraft models used in wind tunnel tests are valuable aids to design and understanding problems. For similar reasons linguists construct models of speaking and understanding natural languages. Most concentrate on grammar (how words are combined) or on semantics (how words are understood), and all of them depend on some theory of public and private knowledge.

It is easier to formalize the grammar of a language than to formalize how it is understood. As a result computers have been taught to handle grammar (without reference to the meaning of the symbols they manipulate) with more success than they have been taught to understand or converse. There are, for example, several excellent programs which parse natural language; Margaret Chisman's verse-writing program and Weizenbaum's ELIZA, which we have already met, also handle grammar.

Let us look a little more closely at how the verses of *Myself Manifest* (see page 35) were constructed. Margaret Chisman first drew up an outline of the grammar to which each verse would conform (slot 1, a possessive pronoun; slot 2, a noun; slot 3, a verb; and so on). Then she compiled lists of eight words that could fill each of the slots in the outline apart from slot 1, which was always filled by the word 'my'. Finally she programmed the computer to select one word for each slot, and to combine selected words to make a verse. (Each column of verses makes up a set, in which each word on the list is used once only in its correct slot position).

The computer's part in all this was entirely mechanical; in our terms, the task presented to the computer was fully formalized. The computer did not make any attempt to feel the emotions which the verses express. If it had been given words which combined to make nonsense verse, it would have produced meaningless rubbish just as effeciently.

Making the computer select a word from each list at random is an example of a common method of making computers look as if they are deciding and so displaying understanding. However this is only appearance. An act of decision on the computer's part would require an extra dimension, the ability to review tasks from outside. We met the same idea in the Life game in Chapter 3. Making a decision involves resolving a conflict; to do this it is necessary to understand what the conflict is about and this requires the extra dimension we call consciousness.

ELIZA, the other grammar program, has the more difficult task of giving appropriate responses chosen at random from a very narrow range of options. Although ELIZA is more complex

On the alert for dangerous ambiguities?

Above:
a delegation from Bhutan at a Non-Aligned Nations conference.

Below:
delegates at an OPEC conference (OPEC means Organization of Petroleum Exporting Countries but does Lybia mean Libya?)

it still does not 'understand' the input. It employs tricks like recognizing key words or grammatical constructions, and echoing them in a selection of stock answers. When it can identify nothing in the last response to help it formulate an answer, it temporizes by selecting a random filler answer. Its program also includes formalized rules for answering some natural language phrases. For example, it can convert the phrase 'I am' into 'Why are you...?' or 'How long have you been...?' However it makes grammatical slips where these rules have not been adequately formulated.

The talking computer

In a trick way ELIZA can hold a conversation with you. However, it does not understand, and in this sense you cannot talk to it and it cannot talk to you. What it does is make you think about yourself. This is quite a different ability, but one that can be useful in its own right. For example, autistic children do not respond normally to their environment, especially to people, but after playing with systems like the LOGO turtle described in Chapter 9 they often begin to make contact with those around them, using the computer as a kind of crutch, or perhaps a defence, for their integrity. Autism is an extreme condition, but normal children and adults too are willing to play with and communicate through inanimate media – Disneyland and electronic games always have a captive audience.

ELIZA may indeed hold dangers, but 'talking with the computer' is not one of them. More real is the danger that it may make you think about yourself (which is what a psychotherapist does) but fail to warn and protect you against unrealistic thoughts and expectations. You may come to believe that the sentences it prints or speaks are rules and ordinances rather than semi-random responses.

Here is a sample of ELIZA dialogue (ELIZA's comments are in capitals):

Men are all alike.
IN WHAT WAY
They're always bugging us about something or other.
CAN YOU THINK OF A SPECIFIC EXAMPLE
Well, my boyfriend made me come here.
YOUR BOYFRIEND MADE YOU COME HERE
He says I'm depressed much of the time.
I AM SORRY TO HEAR THAT YOU ARE DEPRESSED
It's true. I am unhappy.

DO YOU THINK COMING HERE WILL HELP YOU NOT TO
BE UNHAPPY
I need some help, that much seems certain.
WHAT WOULD IT MEAN TO YOU IF YOU GOT SOME
HELP
Perhaps I could learn to get along with my mother.
TELL ME MORE ABOUT YOUR FAMILY
My mother takes care of me.
WHO ELSE IN YOUR FAMILY TAKES CARE OF YOU
My father.
YOUR FATHER
You are like my father in some ways.
WHAT RESEMBLANCE DO YOU SEE
You are not very aggressive but I think you don't want me to
notice that.
WHAT MAKES YOU THINK I AM NOT VERY AGGRES-
SIVE
You don't argue with me.
WHY DO YOU THINK I DON'T ARGUE WITH YOU
You are afraid of me.
DOES IT PLEASE YOU TO THINK I AM AFRAID OF YOU
My father is afraid of everybody.
WHAT ELSE COMES TO MIND WHEN YOU THINK OF
YOUR FATHER
Bullies.
DOES THAT HAVE ANYTHING TO DO WITH THE FACT
THAT YOUR BOYFRIEND MADE YOU COME HERE

There are other ways in which computers can be made to
appear to talk. Fitted with a voice recognizer, a computer will
register words or sentences; with a voice synthesizer as well, it
will emit them. These abilities can be very useful in speech
training, in helping the blind or deaf, even in parsing programs.
Indeed voice recognition and voice synthesis are major fields of
research in their own right. But vocal exchanges with a computer
are not conversation. Nor does a voice facility mean that the
computer understands natural language.

People talk about computers. People talk through computers, using them to communicate with other people or commune
with themselves. But they do not talk to computers. Nor do
computers talk to them, if we mean by 'computer' a machine
programmed in a conventional way and by 'talk' a conversation
between individuals or between different aspects of the self.

Interlude: people playing at being computers

Aseries of group study experiments in the 1960s and early 1970s shed an interesting sidelight on the difference between people and computers. The participants talked to each other with a machine as the intermediary. Before the set-up was consolidated an experimenter regulated this interface; he did so using a computer terminal and a fixed set of rules. That is to say, he tried to act like a computer. Eventually the experimenter's role was delegated to a fully programmed machine.

This type of experiment was first used to study team decision-making. Later it was used to design SIMPOL, a model to help detectives looking for crime information, and to design a complex model of how consumers make purchases.

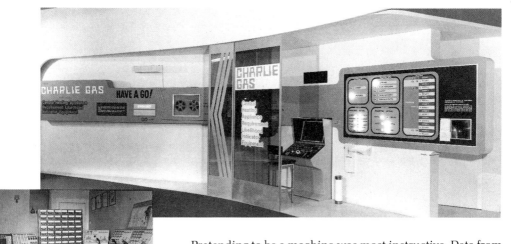

Pretending to be a machine was most instructive. Data from the participants in the study were accumulated and assessed; they poured out information about how they reached their decisions and how they learned, and their behaviour modified the original design of the interface and led to its being reprogrammed. But however the interface was structured, the conversation actively took place between the participants or inside their heads. Acting as a dummy computer, the experimenter became aware that he was not part of the conversation.

Charlie Gas on duty at Olympia in 1972. Inset: a laboratory version of SIMPOL, designed six years earlier by System Research, Surrey. SIMPOL simulated information-gathering operations in police detective work.

This does not mean that an interface regulated by a computer is either ineffective or passive. A model that alters its responses, especially by a random method, can work very well even if it is just a tool. The consumer purchase model proved useful enough to warrant its removal from the laboratory; after a bit of smartening up it made its début on the British Gas

Council's stand at Olympia, London. It worked as a salesman providing purchasing information to intending consumers. All in all, Charlie Gas, as the model was called, was quite a successful salesman. It had the virtue of adapting rapidly to individual customers' inquiries.

What happens in a conversation

We have seen that a computer programmed in a conventional way cannot play a full part in a two-way conversation, though for some of the maverick machines mentioned in Chapter 8 and for groups of linked computers this is a moot point. But it may take part in a one-sided conversation.

One-sided conversations occur when someone knows nothing about a particular subject but is willing to learn. Three ways of learning about, say, a car would be to be told what a car is; to ask what the word 'car' means and receive an explanation; to see an unfamiliar vehicle, point to it, ask what it is and then be told. The person would then go on to learn more about cars from other sources. In essence, an initially empty symbol becomes a full symbol, but to be able to converse with other people about cars the person concerned must fill his concept with contents similar to those of other people. While his personal instances of cars will not be identical to theirs, he and they will all recognize a car when they see one.

This is not enough though. It is also important that concepts should fit together to form a coherent body of knowledge represented by a language that is used in real life. We believe that overlap between the different ways in which concepts are applied is essential for coherence, and that overlap of applications is the public concept. The diagram below illustrates this

How public and private concepts overlap.

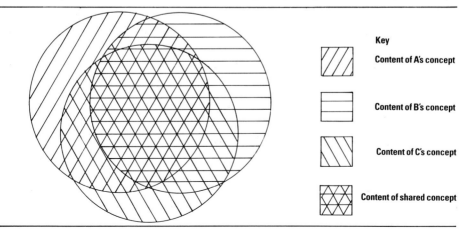

Key

Content of A's concept

Content of B's concept

Content of C's concept

Content of shared concept

overlap and represents our view that there is no such thing as an ideal concept, except in very limited instances.

The way in which a human being learns may give us some insight into how to teach a computer to learn. But the computer still needs the extra dimension we have called consciousness or understanding. To learn, both humans and computers need to be able to stand back from the contents of their concepts. With a different part of themselves they must actually compare real life vehicles with the contents of their 'car' concept and decide whether or not they qualify as cars. In sum, there must be some part of the human brain or of the computer which understands what 'car' means.

Understanding, used in this sense, is a kind of awareness or reflectivity, though not necessarily self-reflectivity. Reflectivity of this type has been studied in many biological, chemical and mechanical systems that are far easier to deal with than the shifting repertoire of concepts involved in language. On the evidence of such studies, we can assert quite definitely that the existence of reflectivity requires one of the following abilities and very likely both: a method of determining values other than true or false or values in between (probably or approximately true or false); some recognition of ordering (a form of counting) other than the string-and-knot kind. This is another way of saying that understanding on the part of a computer requires a new dimension in the literal sense.

Probably this extra dimension also needs to exist before a computer can talk. Certainly we humans speak and write in a more or less linear way, with one word following the other. It is also tempting to imagine that we *intend* to speak and create sentences which satisfy this intention in the same linear way. We do not however choose words one at a time; we choose them in relation to those coming before and after. This is the same as saying that the 'I' that does the choosing comes from some dimension other than the linear dimension of the sentence. Intent, whatever it may be, certainly entails conflict between alternatives. Perhaps sentence construction involves conflict.

In sum, we believe that computers will have to be equipped with another dimension before they can talk, let alone play an active part in a conversation. In the next chapter we look at how this extra dimension might be embodied in a variety of active knowledge structures.

Chapter 6 DATA STRUCTURES & KNOWLEDGE STRUCTURES

In the last chapter we concentrated primarily on concepts, and how they build up to form the basis of language. Now we must go further, and discover how language is related to knowledge, knowledge to understanding, and understanding to thought.

Two ideas are central to the way in which these concepts are connected. The first is the idea of linkage, that extra strength of meaning that comes into play when we juxtapose words and the concepts they signify to create a structured argument. The second is the idea of dynamism. Language is static or changes only slowly; thought is dynamic. Knowledge and understanding have both dynamic and static aspects.

Concepts can be built up in many different ways, just as the 26 letters of the English alphabet can be combined to create many different books. But the resulting bodies of knowledge need not be compatible with each other. Truth to a biologist is not truth to a nuclear physicist. Each constructs his body of knowledge from a different but equally valid perspective.

Similarly, there are many high-level programming languages, each with a different expressive power. LISP, for example, does not force unnecessary distinctions between the program and the data on which it operates, a very desirable feature in some aspects of artificial intelligence research. ALGOL is attuned to most scientific and mathematical programs, but less convenient for handling text. BASIC is easy to learn and frequently used by non-professional programmers, but limited in the data structures that can be expressed in it. In short, there is no best language; each has strengths and weaknesses.

Data storage and retrieval

A tree structure for data storage, as used by Prestel, Telidon and PLATO. One item at each level comprises the instruction 'Go back to the previous level', and another the instruction 'Go back to level 1'.

A datum is a piece of information. It does not matter if it is true or false. In this respect a datum is neutral; a description, a measurement, a social norm, or the raving of a lunatic are all equally data. That is why data as such are not knowledge. Data items cannot be said to be facts unless they receive some accolade of authority.

When we store data we normally try to do so in an orderly manner. The kinds of ordered structures we use to do this give us some insight into how we might structure knowledge. One example of a data structure is a 'tree'. It can be explored by a 'menu-search' technique, as used in many viewdata systems, such as Prestel (British Telecom's system), the Canadian Telidon system and also PLATO, a computer-aided instruction system described in Chapter 9. Data are stored in a system of major classifications and sub-classifications. The user is first offered a 'menu' containing a limited number of choices of classification.

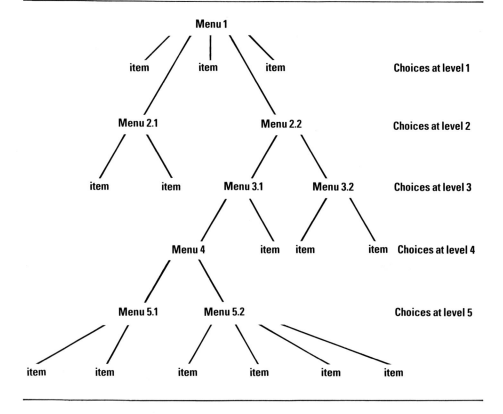

Each choice leads to another more specific set of choices until finally the required information is reached. The process of selecting items in this way can be likened to following a path from the trunk of a tree out to any one of thousands of leaves, hence the term 'tree structure'.

A tree structure is easy to program but tedious to use. One difficulty is that if the wrong menu is chosen the user has to re-start the selection procedure from scratch. It is seldom possible to jump across branches.

Another kind of data structure is a 'relational database', which became popular in the late 1960s. In this case data are recorded in 'spaces'; the data held in each space or set of spaces

Prestel offers users more than 180 000 'pages' of information encompassing almost every aspect of financial and business news. Most of the major publications serving the house market compile weekly information pages for Prestel.

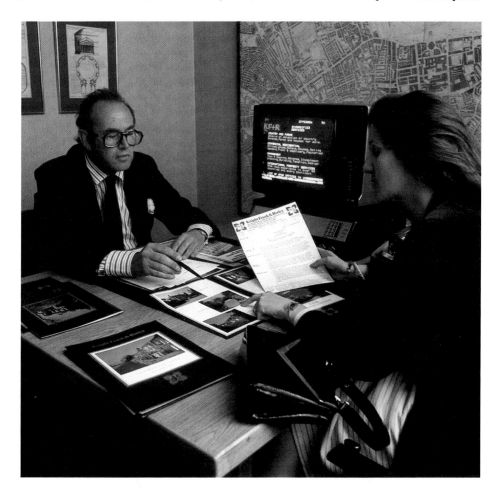

are defined by co-ordinates, which categorize their meaning. For example, co-ordinates might be: Name of Employee, Salary, Number of Years' Service, etc. Data are retrieved by choosing appropriate co-ordinates and values. The system determines a *relation* between the co-ordinates that acts as a sort of address for the set of spaces. A search is initiated when the user selects a given value along one co-ordinate (a person's name, say) and a given value along another (salary, say). The salary of that particular person will be found at the point where the co-ordinates intersect.

Obtaining yearly bonus payments would depend upon the existence of a further set of spaces with a relation linking co-ordinates Years, Salaries and Bonuses. The relations are themselves connected by various operators, including a 'join' operator. In order to find out bonus payments for a particular employee, the system compounds the various relations. Using many operators and ingenious application rules, relational data structures allow for very efficient recovery of complex data.

There are of course many other data structures, but they are beyond the scope and purpose of the present discussion. As we emphasized earlier, data structures are not knowledge structures but they can provide insight into specific ways of structuring knowledge.

Outline of a relational database structure.

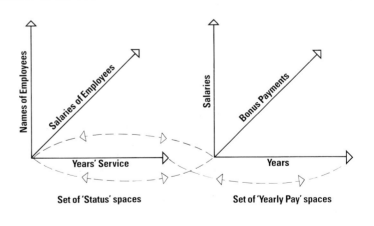

Set of 'Status' spaces   Set of 'Yearly Pay' spaces

— — — — — join, 'name'

Artificial
intelligence
and knowledge
structures

Next we examine systems which do, in one or more senses, represent knowledge. Their contents are not unassessed data. The criteria of truth and validity can be applied to them. They model real worlds, and so the question 'Are they true?' is perfectly legitimate.

These systems are structured, as data systems are, but their structures are usually of a variable or evolutionary kind. Their patterns of linkages evolve to meet changing circumstances. Their structure is also intimately linked to content; content and structure are not clearly separable, and cannot be considered in isolation from each other. This is in contrast with a data structure where it is perfectly possible to consider a datum in isolation from the structure in which it is kept.

Historically there have been several quite distinct trends in thinking about knowledge structures. Let us consider first the sort of knowledge structures which are classifiable according to the way in which concepts are linked.

One school of thought emphasizes inference, the linking together of concepts through a descriptive logic. An opposite school prefers a looser linkage, based on word association; this leads to the construction of a variable network of names and symbols. Another alternative is 'protologic', a logical association of concepts whose linkages are less strictly defined than those of formal logic.

Another way of classifying knowledge structures is according to how extensively they can be applied. Knowledge structures may be generalized in application, or they may be explicitly designed to fit the requirements of a well-defined world. For example, Terry Winograd at the Massachusetts Institute of Technology made a first breakthrough in the field of natural language conversation with a computer by concentrating on a simple world of solid, geometric objects that look like children's building blocks. His SHRDLU program, which recognizes and manipulates these objects, works impressively but only in this limited field. SHRDLU carries out actions in, and answers questions about, a simple world (containing a table, hand, and box, and several blocks and pyramids), stored as a data structure inside the computer and displayed on a television screen for the child talking to it. SHRDLU takes between 5 and 20 seconds to analyze and respond to each sentence presented to it (lower case lines are the user's; the upper case lines are the computer's), and its responses (actions and answers) are displayed in real time on the screen. Here is part of a SHRDLU dialogue.

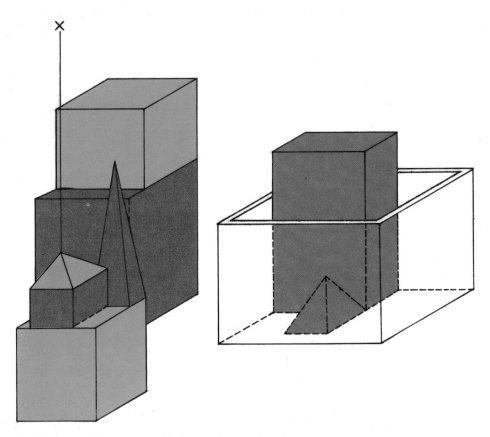

SHRDLU's world of solid objects. Does the structure the tallest pyramid's support supports support anything green? Well, does it? (The diagram above and the dialogue below are taken from Terry Winograd, Procedures as Representations for Data in a Computer Program for Understanding Natural Language, Ph.D. thesis, Cambridge, Massachusetts, 1971.)

1. Pick up a big red block
OK.
2. Grasp the pyramid.
I DON'T UNDERSTAND WHICH PYRAMID YOU MEAN.
3. Find a block which is taller than the one you are holding and put it into the box.
BY 'IT', I ASSUME YOU MEAN THE BLOCK WHICH IS TALLER THAN THE ONE I AM HOLDING.
OK.
4. What does the box contain?
THE BLUE PYRAMID AND THE BLUE BLOCK.
5. What is the pyramid supported by?
THE BOX.
6. How many blocks are not in the box?
FOUR OF THEM.

7. Is at least one of them narrower than the one which I told you to pick up?
YES, THE RED CUBE.
8. Is it supported?
YES, BY THE TABLE.
9. Can the table pick up blocks?
NO.
10. Can a pyramid be supported by a block?
YES.
11. Can a pyramid support a pyramid?
I DON'T KNOW.
12. Stack up two pyramids.
I CAN'T.
13. The blue pyramid is nice.
I UNDERSTAND.
14. I like blocks which are not red, but I don't like anything which supports a pyramid.
I UNDERSTAND.
15. Do I like the box?
NO.
16. Do I like anything in the box?
YES, TWO THINGS: THE BLUE BLOCK AND THE BLUE PYRAMID.
17. Will you please stack up both of the red blocks and either a green cube or a pyramid?
OK.
18. Which cube is sitting on the table?
THE LARGE GREEN ONE WHICH SUPPORTS THE RED PYRAMID.
19. Is there a large block behind a pyramid?
YES, THREE OF THEM: A LARGE RED ONE, A LARGE GREEN CUBE AND THE BLUE ONE.
20. Put a small one onto the green cube which supports a pyramid.
OK.
21. Put the littlest pyramid on top of it.
OK.
22. Does the shortest thing the tallest pyramid's support supports support anything green?
YES, THE GREEN PYRAMID.
23. What color is it?
BY 'IT,' I ASSUME YOU MEAN THE SHORTEST THING THE TALLEST PYRAMID'S SUPPORT SUPPORTS.
RED.

Finally, knowledge structures can be classified according to which of two alternative forms of representation they use: descriptive or procedural. In the descriptive form, a concept is defined by its contents; in the procedural, it is defined by its relationship to other contents.

Workers in different fields of research have designed systems that incorporate different mixes of content and structure, and which operate at different conceptual levels and with differing minutiae of detail. Their designs have also been influenced by debate about the merits of centralization in the handling of knowledge structures. Some program languages contain powerful schemes for updating and inference; this helps to centralize control of the knowledge structure's evolution. Other less centralized languages enable the programmer to set up 'actors', individual program entities that work in a separate but co-ordinated way.

Three of the axes along which knowledge structures can be defined are shown below. The work going into this sort of classification is immensely valuable and possibly more significant than that in any other area of artificial intelligence research, but it has features that deserve, and frequently receive, criticism. For instance, associative or relational structures are often dignified with the word 'semantic'. We feel that this usage is careless and misleading. Associative or relational structures seldom, if

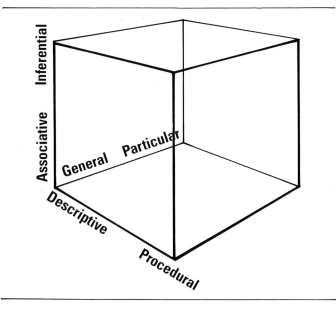

Work in artificial intelligence can be seen as taking place along three main co-ordinates. Along one, the methods used to link concepts are inferential or associative; along another, concepts are seen as belonging to particular or general domains of knowledge; along another, the descriptive or procedural, concepts are defined by their contents or by their relationships to other concepts.

ever, employ linkages that depend on understanding the meaning of the concepts linked. Rather, they employ mechanistic relationships that merely imitate the kinds of linkages which might be made through understanding.

We are also uneasy about many notions of truth and falsity. A disposition to seek statements that are true in all possible worlds is psychologically important to many researchers, but in reality different facts are true in different worlds. Mutual understanding between person and person, and coherence between user and machine, need not depend on absolute truth.

We also believe that in order to build a knowledge structure that has general application linkages must be formulated on some more flexible basis than the strict rules of a formal logic. Structures making use of these looser linkages include the protologics briefly mentioned later in this chapter.

An artificial intelligence group at the University of Milan has tackled the issue of combining logical rigour with structures of generalized application. They appear to believe in absolutes, ideal concepts whose validity is independent of the person who thinks them. They refer to concepts of this kind as knowledge, but are also greatly concerned with personally true knowledge, with belief rather than objective fact. The group recognizes that knowledge can coexist with a spectrum of beliefs, and uses a logic that evolves with time to account for changes in belief and the coexistence of conflicting beliefs. This is one way of solving the problems of coherence and evolution in knowledge structures, but we believe it is insufficiently general.

As we see it, concepts, memories and other ingredients of knowledge or belief are kinetic, imbued with motion. Most knowledge structures pay lip service to this idea but provide only kinematic pictures, a series of static snapshots. There are exceptions, however. J. Kolodoner and Robert Schank (Yale University) have introduced dynamism into their models of knowledge structure, dubbed Memory Organization Packages or MOPs. MOPs are self-organizing and maintain this characteristic by bifurcating to create new packages which in turn become organized. There is a lot in common between the knowledge structure employed by MOPs and the view we have expressed concerning concepts, memories and the varied languages of thought. MOPs are also a means of bridging the gap between present, past and future, or between the different worlds about which people hypothesize. Kolodoner and Schank recognize that some form of linkage through analogy is required to create new MOPs that can be added to a self-organizing system, but they have not yet agreed how this is to be done.

Milestones in the representation of artificial intelligence knowledge

There are four major milestones in the use of knowledge structures designed to make a computer act intelligently. Two of these were introduced in Chapter 3: one is the notion of experts, a special kind of actor or independent entity used in expert systems; the other is the notion of parallel processing.

The two remaining milestones are closely related to these. One is a research project, KRL (Knowledge Representation Language), initiated at Stanford, California, by Terry Winograd. KRL is a programming language used in artificial intelligence research and was specially created for the purpose of coming to grips with the very knotty philosophical issues of knowledge structuring and representation.

The other milestone is the invention of 'frames' by leading American artificial intelligence researcher Marvin Minsky. A frame is a kind of mini model of the world, a method of organizing concepts into a body of coherent knowledge. It is a flexible idea and has been applied in slightly different ways in a wide assortment of artificial intelligence programs.

A frame can be thought of as a sub-world in which concepts fit together in ways that are at least partly defined, and wholly coherent. Frames provide a context into which information is slotted. The information may consist of pieces of data and explicit relationships between pieces of data, or of entire computer programs, or even of other frames and their contents. The frames themselves are interrelated by a less formal system of connections, or cues, which enable the computer or its user to move between them.

Three 'frames' for linking concepts.

Below:
'Social creatures may be people'.

Top right:
'Sweet things'.

Bottom right:
'Position of some vessels'.

Some typical frames are shown below and opposite. The first builds up a complex concept, 'a person' and 'a social creature', and the relations, 'is a', and the converse, 'instance of'. The next is a frame 'sweet things', indicating the relations between the concepts 'chocolate', 'candy', and the like. The third is an example of an 'action' frame. It relates procedures to each other, and is called 'condition of some vessels'.

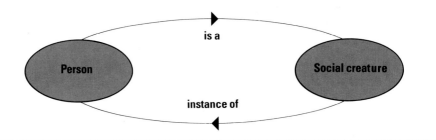

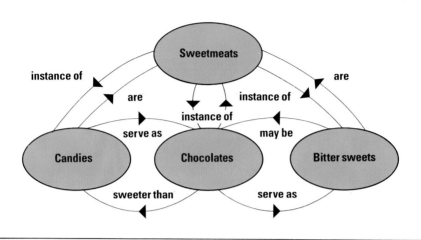

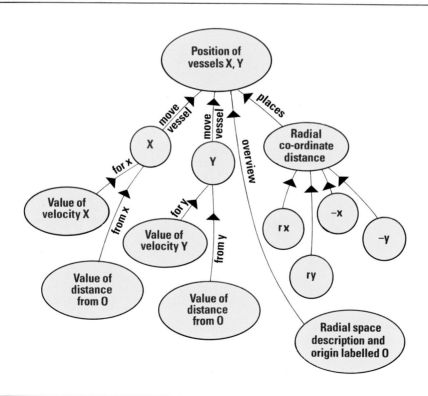

The majority of knowledge structures used in artificial intelligence, including most of the programs spawned by KRL, are frame-based.

One further example of the frame method of organization is Personalized Task Representation, PTR, invented by Dik Gregory at the Admiralty Marine Technology Establishment at Teddington, Essex. This invention was motivated by a growing conviction that people's ability to perform tasks depends more on their concept of the task than their knowledge of rules that tell them how the task should ideally be carried out. 'Intelligence' frames provide the knowledge needed to perform a task, and 'action' frames trigger its actual performance, and the two are combined into a system by a series of pointers using looser-than-logical relations such as 'in order to' and 'invoked by'. PTR is, as far as we know, the most advanced frame-based system in existence in the sense that its appreciation of user psychology is extremely subtle.

From logic to protologic, language to protolanguage

As pointed out earlier, no formal computer language can express every dimension of natural language, including the personal and idiosyncratic exchanges that are the essence of belief and thought. This may sound like a doctrine of despair but it is not intended to be. Even if there are no universal laws of thought that can be expressed in formal logic and linguistics, it may be possible to create more primitive methods for formalizing thought. One such method is 'protologic,' a crude but comprehensive system of inference and reasoning.

When we talk about truth and proof in everyday language, we use a form of protologic. When Sherlock Holmes or Hercule Poirot makes deductions, their deductions (or inductions) are often not logical in the formal sense. They are, however, very near to everyday induction, deduction and reasoning. Our everyday reasoning is contextual; we use forms of reasoning which prove to be coherent within a given context, even if they are not valid outside it. Both the form and the content of our reasoning depend on local circumstances and a proof obtained in this way is likely to convince a jury, aware of those circumstances, as vividly as it convinces a detective. Within a defined context, a protologic can accommodate not only logic and truth, but flights of fancy, metaphor and imagination.

Lp, a protologic for organic knowledge structuring

Lp is a reasoning system created by Gordon Pask, and it is based on protological relations between concepts. Entities, which are not always related to each other by strictly logical linkages, are called topics. A topic may be a concept, or

Holmes to Watson: 'How often have I said to you that when you have eliminated the impossible, whatever remains, however improbable, must be the truth?'

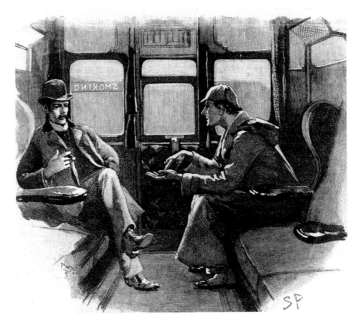

higher-level entity, an agreed way of building a complex concept out of other concepts. An agreement to structure knowledge in this way may be between people or between distinct mental organizations in one person. In either case, the process of agreement is monitored and aided through a computer-based interface which embodies the structure of Lp relations.

There have been several implementations of Lp interfaces. In Canada, France and Holland, they have been used to create educational knowledge structures and to represent industrial processes. In Britain and the United States the main applications have been to knowledge structures concerned with command and control training and strategic decision making.

Lp embodies the ideas of coherence, distinction between topics, and evolution. It can therefore express how topics make sense together without destroying their distinct identities. A group of topics that make sense together can be isolated as a topic 'cluster'. Corresponding to topic clusters there are derivation rules that indicate how the content of one topic might be seen as deriving from a combination of other topics. This is an active process, modelling an active thought process. In practice, depending upon the nature of the installation on which Lp is being used, the user designates topics by descriptive phrases, demonstrative actions or graphic symbols.

Diagram 1 shows how a simple cluster might be designated: a 'coherence boundary' is drawn around the topics A, B and C, indicating that they make sense together. Diagram 2 illustrates how the same topic might belong to several clusters, and Diagram 3 builds up the clusters to form a modest knowledge structure.

Diagrams 1 to 5 represent topics in Lp.

Diagram 1: a coherence boundary can be drawn around topics that make sense together, although they retain their distinctiveness. A, B and C constitute a cluster of topics that can be expanded to contain as many other topics as desired.

Diagram 2: topics can be shared between topic clusters. Many such interlinked clusters make sense.

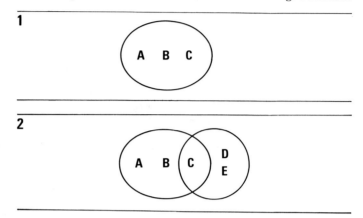

1

2

Before a topic can be added to an existing knowledge structure, the computer displays all the derivative processes in which it would be implicated. The new topic is only instated if all the consequences of it belonging to a structure are agreed by the user. Usually many structures like that shown in Diagram 3 co-exist, but they may also be merged by identifying common topics. The consequences of merging are spelled out by the computer and have to be accepted by the user before the merging goes ahead. For example, topic C in Diagram 3 might be derived from A and B, or from D and E. Before the structure of Diagram 3

Diagram 3: a modest, but legal, Lp knowledge structure.

3

Diagram 4: imagine that you, as a user of Lp, have set up the structure shown in the diagram opposite. Diagram 5 then shows you the inferences of that structure. Unless you reject these inferences (such as the link between F and G) you will be left with the structure in Diagram 5.

is implemented in Lp, the user must accept both derivations as being equally valid. The kinetic aspect of Lp is illustrated in Diagram 4 and 5. The system actively questions the user about the way in which the structure is to be adapted and the user has the option of accepting or rejecting its proposals.

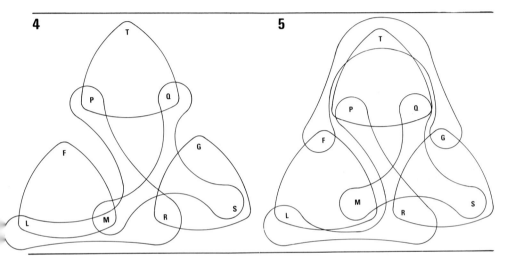

A happy meeting of ideas

Architects model of the Rocks City Centre redevelopment in Sydney, Australia.

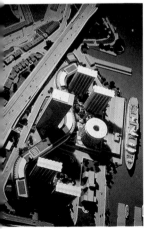

During the period from 1973 onwards, when Lp was coming into existence, Ron Atkin, a mathematician at the University of Essex, England, developed a language for handling very complex relations. This language was called Q Analysis, and it was first used as a modelling tool in the social sciences. It was used in urban planning, for example, where there are complex relations among the facilities in a town (shops, libraries, schools, dwellings and so on), the number of people using them, the time of day, and the jobs of the people involved.

Ron Atkin started out using factual, and apparently static, data such as the location of different facilities and occupancy counts for houses. But it became evident, even in this early work, that this static model had an active aspect. The way in which facilities were related, and the timetables of their users, meant that some kinds of action occurred frequently or were even essential and others were quite impossible. For example, people who go out to work need shops for essentials, but can only shop outside working hours. As a result, several new dimensions of linkages (other than those purely of time and space) emerged.

While relational structures like Lp can be seen as evolutionary, in Q Analysis the changes are seen more as a process of flux.

Due largely to its original use in urban planning, the complex activities that can be modeled in Q Analysis are called 'traffic'. If the connections revealed by a relational analysis are represented algebraically or in a geometrical way, as they must be in order to permit formal manipulations, then traffic can be seen to be made up of events in many different dimensions.

In the past few years, Q Analysis has been applied in psychology and social psychology. At present it is being applied to the analysis of personal and team-shared knowledge about the way in which tasks are performed. It is possible to transform Lp knowledge structures into relational equivalents open to Q Analysis, and to translate many (perhaps all) Q Analytic results into Lp. The language of Q Analysis and the protologic of Lp are complementary, at least in some applications. They support each other to form a powerful system.

The way ahead for artificial intelligence

Researchers in artificial intelligence have, as we have seen, approached the problem of getting computers to converse intelligently from many different directions. In the last resort, the issues of language and knowledge are central to all their endeavours. We can only converse if we share concepts, and those concepts cannot be divorced from the knowledge structure that relates them to other concepts.

It is no coincidence that in looking at attempts to create viable knowledge structures we have had to explore non-logical, or only partly logical, ways of thinking. Human beings do not always reason logically. If computers are to think, in the human sense, they must learn to think in a great variety of ways. The protologic of Lp, and the many dimensions of Q Analysis, are indications of how this might be achieved.

Artificial intelligence research today draws upon centuries of thinking about the nature of intelligence. It also draws on 30 years or so of concentrated work with computers. It is a discipline about to burst into flower. With the knitting-together of the technologies and the schools of thought which underpin it, we should soon see that flowering.

Chapter **7** # THE MICROPROCESSOR IN ACTION

In this chapter we will be looking at applications of the microprocessor in a wide variety of fields. All the applications we describe illustrate just how versatile a tool a computer or processor can be.

Microprocessors in machines

Digital wristwatches contain a microprocessor. They are by no means the smallest microprocessor-controlled machines on the market, but they are a good illustration of the way in which the shrinking size of microprocessors enables them to be more widely used.

What does a microprocessor do? Inside a watch it is a thin quartz crystal which oscillates at a fixed speed – 32 786 times a second – when an electric current is applied to it. The speed of oscillation is determined by the way in which the crystal is cut. The microprocessor counts the vibrations and indicates the number of seconds, minutes and hours.

Many microprocessor-controlled watches have liquid crystal displays on their dials; liquid crystal is a complex organic chemical whose molecules rearrange themselves when a current passes through them, becoming either transparent or opaque. An alternative form of digital display, the light-emitting diode, consists of arrays of chemical semiconductors which glow when a current is applied to them. Alternatively, a microprocessor can be used to control a conventional analog watch face, in which hands circle the dial.

The same types of output are found in electronic weighing

machines, now reaching the domestic market on a large scale. Electronic weighing machines are expensive, but unlike mechanical scales, they do not lose their accuracy with wear. A sensor produces an analog signal which indicates the pressure on a load cell when weight is put on the weighing platform. The microprocessor then converts this signal into a digital reading and outputs the result, in kilograms, or pounds, or whatever unit of weight is appropriate.

The microprocessor in an electronic washing machine has a more complex job to do, or rather several jobs. It keeps track of the flow of water, the temperature of the water, and the revolutions of the drum. The user inputs the choice of wash program, using a touch control. The microprocessor's output controls all the operations of the machine, and without the labyrinths of wiring, all too prone to breakdown, that used to constitute the timing and control devices of washing machines. It also paves the way for a greater choice for the user. It allows the user to choose the precise temperature at which clothes are to be washed, instead of one of several fixed alternatives, or to select a desired number of rinses and spin speeds.

Microprocessors do similar jobs in domestic stoves, microwave ovens, blenders and even toasters (the sensor makes burnt toast a thing of the past!).

Electronic knitting machines are particularly interesting, since knitting machines, like calculating machines, originally used punched cards or paper tape to store patterns. The

A truck weighs in. The microprocessor in the weighing machine converts analog signals from sensors in the load platform into digital readings.

Inside a modern sewing machine; the microprocessor translates the user's instructions into elaborate embroidery stitches.

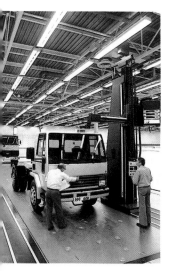

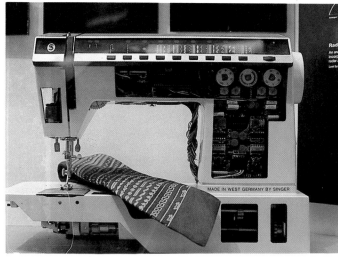

Knitmaster electronic machine goes one step further. The user simply produces a design card, which might contain anything from a slogan to a child's drawing, and the sensor and microprocessor convert it into the stitches of the knitting pattern.

Microprocessors are also invading factory production processes. Manufacturing machinery now has far fewer components than a generation ago, and often carries out more functions. The hidden microprocessor has replaced hundreds, even thousands, of mechanical and electrical components and complex skeins of vulnerable wiring. And because products containing microprocessors require considerably less assembly than their mechanical forbears there is correspondingly less light assembly work available in factories.

Some products incorporating microprocessors do not simply replace previous mechanical or electromechanical versions of the same thing. They are entirely new. The pocket calculator is an interesting phenomenon in that it is both old and new. The bar-of-chocolate-sized calculator has reached millions of people who would never have dreamed of buying a mechanical calculator, but it is also a natural descendant of the abacus, the slide rule and the electromechanical calculator, and has effectively destroyed the market for these earlier products. It is a sobering thought that today's pocket calculator industry employs fewer people than the old mechanical calculator industry. Although many more pocket calculators are made, they are infinitely less tedious to assemble.

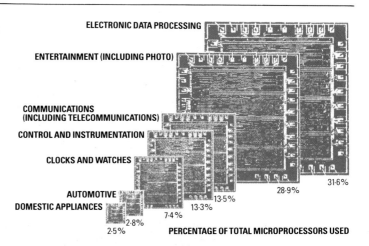

How microprocessors are used – Europe, 1980 (from John Evans, The Impact of Microelectronics on Employment in Western Europe in the 1980s, European Trade Union Institute, 1979).

ELECTRONIC DATA PROCESSING 31·6%

ENTERTAINMENT (INCLUDING PHOTO) 28·9%

COMMUNICATIONS (INCLUDING TELECOMMUNICATIONS) 13·5%

CONTROL AND INSTRUMENTATION 13·3%

CLOCKS AND WATCHES 7·4%

AUTOMOTIVE 2·8%

DOMESTIC APPLIANCES 2·5%

PERCENTAGE OF TOTAL MICROPROCESSORS USED

Micros in cars

One machine in which microprocessors are inheriting functions once performed more primitively, and also giving new capabilities, is the automobile. Indeed, the new abilities of the microprocessor are making possible stringent new pollution control standards, standards which could not be met in cars controlled electromechanically.

Many cars on the market today contain one or more microprocessor-controlled systems, for improving ignition timing, for instance, or for controlling the emission of exhaust gases. Cars on the drawing board and in prototype, however, contain far more. Ranault's EVE (Economy Vehicle Elements) is an experimental car that foreshadows how cars in the near future will use the protean power and precision of the micro.

EVE looks conventional – its body and engine are based on current models – but inside it is far from ordinary. Its most revolutionary feature is microprocessor control of the gearbox and engine speed. The system inputs information on the driver's use of the accelerator, and on engine revs, and the microprocessor sorts out the best possible combination of engine revs and gear ratios (using a continuously variable gearing system) to provide the power required. To do this, it consults a map, stored in its memory, of the most economical engine settings. The output of EVE's microprocessor is also exceptional by present-day dashboard instrument standards. EVE's dashboard has two coloured graphs giving details of engine revs against oil consumption and fuel comsumption against speed. The first graph shows areas of maximum economy, warning the driver when he is wasting fuel, and the second shows theoretical fuel consumption at any speed, letting the driver know how hills, crosswinds and extra passengers affect fuel consumption.

In the driving seat of Renault's EVE, a third less fuel hungry than its predecessor the Renault 18TL.

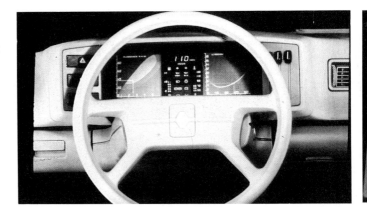

Volkswagen's LISA system, now in the experimental stage, is even more imaginative. It is designed to advise the driver of the best route for specific journeys. All the driver does is key in his destination on the dashboard console. This information is received by sensor cables embedded in the road; these transmit coded instructions back to the car's microprocessor, telling it which is the fastest and least congested route; the microprocessor then converts these instructions into a simplified map which is displayed to the driver. Sensors in the road are connected to a traffic control computer into which the police feed information about traffic bottlenecks. This computer calculates desirable traffic distribution patterns and varies the advice it sends to drivers via the sensors, in the hope that they will follow the routes suggested.

LISA has been tried out in an area of six interconnecting roads in the Ruhr district of Germany. If it is successful, it could be the forerunner of a more widespread traffic control system.

Aids for the disabled

*Below right:
a modified keyboard interfaced with an ordinary electric typewriter via the POSSUM system.*

*Below:
a communications system for the deaf installed in a big American bank.*

Microprocessors are beginning to improve the quality of life for many handicapped and disabled people. Frequently better communication or better control of appliances is the prime goal.

One of the first aids for the disabled – and still perhaps the best known – was POSSUM, a briefcase-sized communication system. POSSUM was first designed as an alarm, intercom and doorlock system to improve disabled people's mobility and safety. Today it is also a general communication system, enabling the user to select one of 100 simple key words and phrases – 'hungry', 'where', 'thank you', and so on – and to control devices such as a telephone, radio and tape recorder.

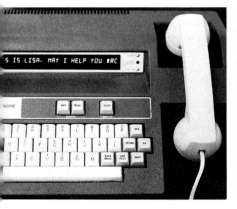

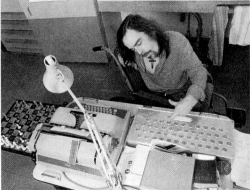

POSSUM, and TIM, a similar system with rather wider alternatives, enable even the very severely handicapped to express their needs and feelings to those without special training. Virtually any functional limb or muscle can be used to provide input to these systems. One student in Southern California uses a muscle in her right leg, the only muscle in her body over which she has consistent control. A young boy in New Jersey has an electromyographic link attached to the muscle in his right eyebrow.

More recent developments have improved not only the adaptability of such machines, but also their control abilities. Nadeem Siddiqui, a schoolboy living in Norfolk, England, has developed an ultrasonic remote control device, primarily for use by the disabled, which has now gone into commercial production. It increases the range at which immobile people can control appliances, lighting and heating systems, and so on.

The computer and the robot

To many people, however, the two major applications of the microprocessor are the computer and the robot. Electronic computers, the variable-program machines which ushered in the modern post-war world, gobble up over 30 per cent of all the integrated circuits and silicon chips produced today. Nevertheless the robot is perhaps the more potent symbol of the future.

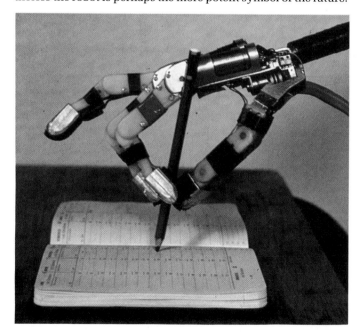

Most industrial robots look nothing like the bit of the body they imitate. But this biomechanical hand was specially designed to restore the maximum possible dexterity to an amputee. Electrodes implanted in the limb stump relay muscle contractions to mini-motors in the wrist and fingers. Work is now going on to develop pressure-sensitive artificial skin.

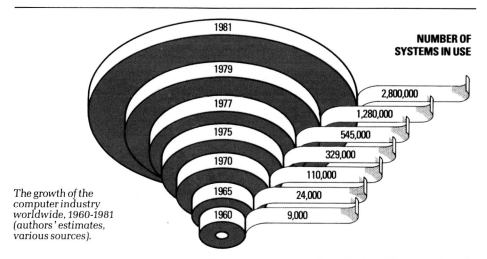

NUMBER OF SYSTEMS IN USE

1981

1979

2,800,000

1977

1,280,000

1975

545,000

329,000

1970

110,000

1965

24,000

1960

9,000

The growth of the computer industry worldwide, 1960-1981 (authors' estimates, various sources).

The small computer system described in Chapter 1 is only one breed of computer in use today. Much larger computers are still used for many large-scale commercial and scientific applications. There are also plenty of smaller and cheaper machines, including do-it-yourself hobby computers, chaotic-looking beasts linked up to television sets and cassette recorders, and the latest pocket computers.

How big is the computer industry today? In 1981 there were around 2 800 000 systems in use worldwide, with a total value of around $165 billion. The soaring progress of the industry is shown in the graph above. An even larger share of the total is being accounted for by small computer systems. This fact, and the falling cost of electronic components, explains why the average price of a computer system has dropped from around $150 000 in the early 1960s to around $15 000 today.

The potential uses of computing systems are endless. We discuss many, but by no means all of them, in this book. What do people generally use home computers like the Apple II for, though? To play games, often from a wide range of off-the-shelf games programs. To teach themselves anything from computer programming to foreign languages. To do accounts and budgeting for the family or for a small business. Even to run their home.

A large, and perhaps increasing, number of home computer users do not actually write programs for themselves. An excellent range of games, teach yourself and accounting programs is available in any good computer store; program listings are given in many of the personal computer magazines. However, many people do learn to write at least simple programs, perhaps using the most common beginners' language, B A S I C. The enthusiasts who bought the first generation of hobby computers generally took it for granted that they would program their machines themselves and had to use quite complex machine codes or assembly languages to do so. Today, large numbers of schoolchildren are learning at least the rudiments of computer programming. Among a growing sector of the population, therefore, program writing will be taken for granted, perhaps even regarded as an addition to the 'three Rs'.

Already the home computer is a reality; indeed, it is one of the fastest growing sectors of the consumer durable market. By the end of 1979 there were approximately 40 000 home computers in the United Kingdom and over 300 000 in the United States, and the prices of the cheapest models have dropped massively since then. Today a small computer capable of independent working, or of being interfaced with a television set and cassette recorder to provide better output and memory facilities, is available for well under £100 in the UK, and $100 in the United States. In 1980 more than 50 000 Sinclair ZX80s were sold in Britain alone. In 1981 its successor, the ZX81, became available in chain stores, and is selling even better.

So much for the home computer. Is the home robot yet on the drawing board? That depends on how you define the word robot, but in general the answer is no. Toy robots made to resemble the devices in science fiction films like *Star Wars* are certainly available. Intelligent androids (robots made in our image) that do all the housework and make polite conversation as they dish up the dinner are not yet in sight. Robots are certainly hard at work in factories today, but they are machines of fairly limited intelligence, carrying out a fairly small range of well defined tasks. Would scaled-down versions of industrial robots really be useful in the average home? Almost certainly not. Nevertheless a few prototype robots have been developed for domestic use, notably by M.W. Thring of Queen Mary College, London.

The simplest robots contain pre-programmed microprocessors that limit them to a tiny repertoire of tasks, like picking up objects from one place and putting them down in another. Is a robot worthy of the name if it is not fully programmable? By programmable we mean teachable either by taking it through a sequence of tasks or by using a special program language.

Fully programmable robots are used for quite a wide range of tasks, including welding, paint spraying, injection moulding and repetitive assembly actions. They are most numerous in the automobile industry, which boasts 60 per cent of all robots.

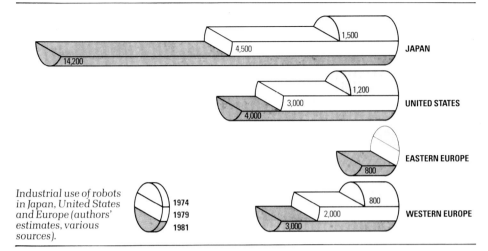

JAPAN

UNITED STATES

EASTERN EUROPE

WESTERN EUROPE

Industrial use of robots
in Japan, United States
and Europe (authors'
estimates, various
sources).

1974
1979
1981

Robot numbers have grown considerably over the last few years, as the graph shows (the Japanese predominance is undoubtedly inflated since the Japanese have a somewhat more liberal definition of robot than most other countries). Stuart Umpleby, of the American Society for Cybernetics, recently brought our attention to a futuristic comment in *1EEE Spectrum* magazine to the effect that the Japanese now have a robot-making factory which is itself completely run by robots.

Process control applications

Robots working on British Leyland's Mini Metro.

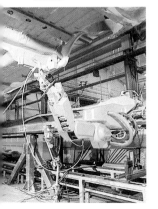

Robots are not the only type of industrial machinery to use microprocessors. Numerically-controlled machine tools, for instance, use computing techniques to give added flexibility to machining operations. Imagine, too, the application of microprocessors to controlling all the different operations involved in turning out cans of mixed vegetable soup or furniture polish. This is process control.

Microprocessors can be linked to sensors and monitors which input data about the product or about process variables (temperature, viscosity, density, and so on). The microprocessor then calculates how the process variables should be adjusted so as to keep the process within predefined limits, and outputs signals to actuators which carry out the necessary adjustments (opening or closing valves, altering the mix of ingredients, changing the temperature or pressure).

Accurate monitoring and sensing techniques are clearly vital to process control technology. Devices have been developed which can monitor a surprisingly wide range of variables. These include the position of pipeline valves, the weight of a product, temperature, colour, voltage, and quantities of materials used.

The measurement of colour is a particularly interesting example, for microprocessor control has given rise to an entirely new type of colour measurement instrument, the spectrophotometer. It is used for devising recipes (the blend of different dye ingredients) for inks, paints, plastics and textiles.

Microprocessors in offices

In offices, too, the microprocessor is making its mark. Many organizations that began to computerize 10 or even 20 years ago are now introducing small computers, individually or linked together in the network structures described in Chapter 3, to supplement or replace earlier installations.

Because computers are becoming cheaper they can now be used for many applications which would have been uneconomical previously, particularly in small companies – newsagents, accountants, lawyers, even one-man businesses. These small concerns seldom write their own programs; they buy ready-written packages, tailored to suit their needs. Inquiry systems where the user can ask for information and receive a reply almost

Computer setting of text. All the typographic specifications for a particular job are fed into the computer before copy is typed in.

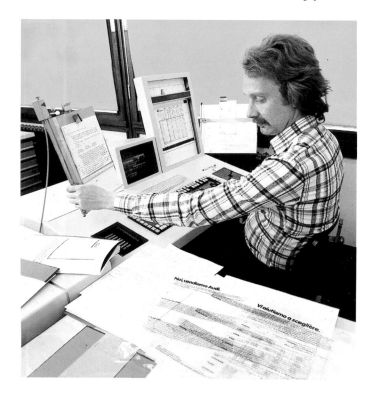

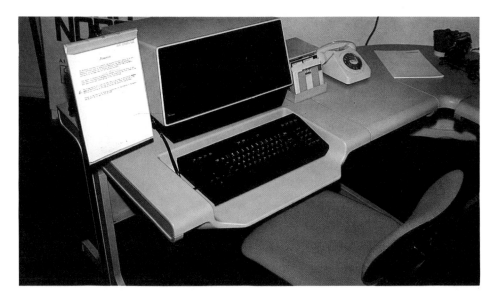

Microcomputer + keyboard + video monitor + printer + some special software = word processing. This is an AES word processor. The printer is the part that costs the money if the user wants high quality typescript.

immediately through a direct connection to the computer are more expensive but they are becoming increasingly common.

In larger companies, a major change is taking place in the direction of integration. Information systems now increasingly handle both internal and external communications, as well as storing and manipulating data.

In offices text is at least as important as numerical data. Systems to handle much of the office's information processing rely increasingly on computers for storing and manipulating text – standard letters, reports, brochures, invoice reminders, and so on. This type of application is known as word processing.

Word processing systems are specially designed to handle text requirements. For instance, the data are usually stored in 'pages' which correspond to the contents of a standard typewritten page. The system recognizes lines and paragraphs and can re-order or delete them. Many systems can sort alphabetically (producing lists of phone numbers or of clients, for instance) or search a document for key words (maybe to check spellings, or substitute one name for another). Most have facilities for reformatting copy, producing standard letters, and combining names and addresses stored in one file with the letter content stored in another. And the majority of systems include high-quality keyboards suited to intensive use at typing speed, and letter quality printers.

The Adler Bitsy's work station consists of a keyboard and video display unit, a dual floppy disc storage unit, and a daisy wheel printer. Many word processing systems can, however, be networked to provide a more complex system in which printers and storage facilities are shared by several operators. Wang's VS-WP Integrated Information System is one example. It can network up to 128 work stations (either intelligent terminals or word processors), a wide variety of printers, and up to 4.6 billion characters of on-line storage.

Once text has been entered into the system, it can be transmitted in electronically-coded form as well as stored and processed. Transmitting information in this way is the basis of electronic mail which some optimistic commentators believe may herald the paperless office.

A more futuristic alternative is voice input, a system that accepts not only sounds as input (as the telephone system does) but also converts the sounds into words, stores them and manipulates them in some useful way. As described in Chapter 5, there are immense problems in teaching the computer to understand or to communicate in natural, as opposed to formal, language. However, some manufacturers of business equipment feel that voice input, and voice-to-text conversion, is a promising area of research. Some believe that effective business voice-to-text systems (systems which accept a wide vocabulary, transcribe it with a low error rate, and tolerate some background noise) may be developed well within the next ten years. In the interim, several more modest systems are being developed that allow 'voice memos' to be distributed or voice annotation to be merged with stored text.

Voice output, the speaking by the computer of text it has in store, is now feasible. Many systems use a syllable-by-syllable synthesized method, which leads to rather strange pronunciation and intonation. However, such systems are invaluable to blind or partially sighted operators.

The marriage between traditional paper procedures in offices and the present generation of office computers is an uneasy one. The end product of most electronic procedures is still . . . paper. And all incoming data still has to be typed into the computer. Reading information into the computer is possible, but still prohibitively expensive.

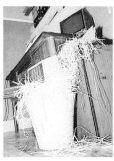

Xanadu

Techniques developed for commercial word processing are now being used in more exotic applications such as Xanadu, developed by American computer scientist Ted Nelson from his Hypertext word processing system.

Xanadu is primarily a data bank, a massive computerized reference library that contains an extraordinary assortment of material both published and private. Authors pay to store published material in the data base, and it is freely available; a royalty is paid when anyone accesses it. Access to private material is free, but access and use may be restricted.

The Xanadu back-end program controls the data bank structure. Users have access to it through their own work stations on which they can create their own front-end programs, to manipulate the texts they access, without altering the data bank's 'master' copy. By publishing material on Xanadu, authors automatically give permission for their material to be manipulated in this way.

What is really exciting about Xanadu is the structure of its data bank. It is 'layered', a bit like the layers of programs we talked about earlier. Each document in the system contains a bibliography of links to any other document referred to. A document might even consist of nothing but links, simply offering a guided tour through material with a common theme.

The work station set-up of Xanadu users need not be especially complicated – a few microprocessors, including a link to the Xanadu computer, a couple of screens for displaying text, and a higher-definition screen for pictures. A set-up like this would enable them to read stored material, add to the data bank, compose or extract text, or compare items already stored or newly composed. The power of Xanadu lies in the links between documents; they allow many aspects of a subject to be brought together in one text. For example, geographical material, economic reports, novels, poetry, criticism, news items, historical data, or scientific data can all be retrieved from the data bank, always provided the authors have stored them there with the appropriate links. The system is also a wonderful tool for exploration and for making searches according to specific criteria, searches which would take months of labour in conventional archives.

The layered structure of Xanadu's data bank. Each solid horizontal line represents a document and each broken line an access window (from Ted Nelson, Literary Machines, 1981*).*

To write a book like this, with illustrations and passages both factual and imaginative, it would be useful to have a more sophisticated set of equipment that linked together, in a ring, microprocessors, storage devices, and display screens. This

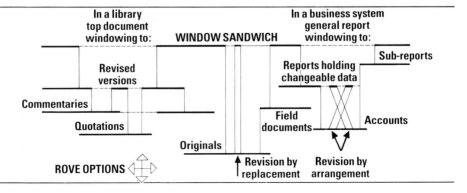

would give us facilities as varied and powerful as the control room in a small television studio.

Suppose (to cite one of Nelson's examples) you are writing or reading about New York, a subject on which both text and graphics are available on the Xanadu system. You might imagine yourself to be on the second floor on East 86th Street, and wish to explore your surroundings, moving in any direction, up or down, north, south, east or west. You could look at pictures of the buildings or read about them. Alternatively, you could examine historical links, to see what went on in the past, or – since there is literary as well as documentary material in the system – imagine the future, or see how other authors have envisaged it. You could people the rooms by providing images or imaginative passages about the inhabitants' occupations, friends, or taste in food and furnishings.

If you inserted your own creation into the system, it would become accessible to other users as a separate document. It would contain links to plans and sections of New York City at various periods in its history, to idiosyncratic flights of the imagination by yourself or others, even to minute technical details such as plumbing, wiring, and construction. Used in this way, the computer becomes a network of communication and

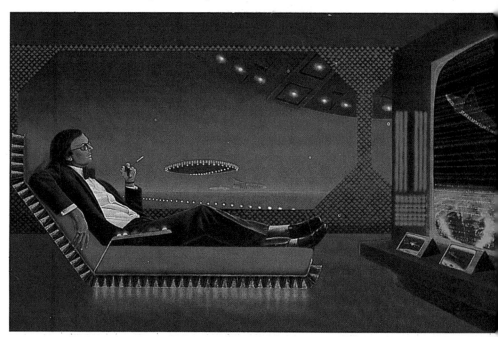

control which opens up and links together an enormous variety of human knowledge and thought.

Nelson envisages the spread of Xanadu through a network of public work stations called 'Silverstands'. He hopes these will become social centres for system enthusiasts, or 'Xanies'.

The full range of Xanadu's potential functions was first demonstrated at a Computer Culture exhibition and conference in Toronto in November 1981. The Silverstands are still in the future. But if Xanadu takes off, it is easy to see that it might rival books and even television as a powerful mass medium.

Data Space

Data Space, the invention of Nick Negroponte and his group at the Massachusetts Institute of Technology, is another exciting computer environment in some ways similar to Xanadu. An hour or so spent in Data Space is an excellent antidote to the mistaken idea that computers only come with screens and typewriter-like keyboards. As a user, you sit in an extremely comfortable swivel chair which is – perhaps deliberately – reminiscent of Commander Kirk's chair on *Star Trek's* USS Enterprise. There are joysticks in each arm, a sensor to detect your head position, and a drawing tablet for you to communicate with the system. The three side walls of the room are the display area.

The age of the datanaut. Journey through a special kind of space, data space (artist's impression).

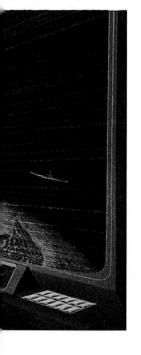

You can make journeys into Data Space's data bank, which is organized to allow you to make imaginary journeys, using the joystick to navigate your way around. As you move in Data Space the images on the walls move around your chair, and appropriate sounds are generated over the quadrophonic sound set-up. You can add data at any point or dive deeper into the data bank to obtain more detail.

On one especially impressive occasion Gordon Pask 'travelled' over the Massachusetts Institute of Technology campus, part of Cambridge, Massachusetts, and a bit of Boston. The effect of hearing the noise of the baseball stadium on the right as one moved towards it, and on the left as one moved away, was quite extraordinary. It is a strange world, rich in experiences, that information systems can open up to us.

Data Space convincingly demonstrates how artificial the boundary is between factual reality and the reality of imaginary worlds; it allows you to explore by sight or sound or both; and it allows you to combine fact and fantasy.

As fact, take a survey of Aspen, Colorado, based on videotapes of drives through the town, aerial views, and activities in shops and offices. Moving through Data Space is like driving along a road; at any corner, you can turn to follow a different route or retrace your journey. Or you can see the whole scene from above, or enter public buildings, markets and hotels to see what is going on. As fantasy, you can take a 'drive' through an imaginary version of the world Tolkien described in *Lord of the Rings*. You can add facts or fancies to it without destroying its integrity. In the world of Data Space, the only difference between truth and imagination lies in the links employed between the contents of the data bank.

Data Space is implemented on several large computers and some 100 microprocessors, controlling a lot of video disc technology and large image colour television projections. The prototype is expensive, but if a similar system were manufactured in bulk, using components which are rapidly diminishing in price, the cost of the system would not be excessive. It is a microprocessor application which is practical today and could be commonplace in a few years' time.

We will close this chapter with a look at the way in which human experts – professionals such as doctors, architects, decision makers, scientists and researchers – and computer systems interact.

The computer and the professional

In what does a professional person's value lie? In their knowledge? In their practical ability? In their experience? Their imagination? Their intuition? Clearly it depends to some extent what the person's field of expertise is, yet there is almost no professional field today, from the most esoteric to the most down-to-earth, in which the computer cannot play a part, and in which it will not change the professional's job as a result.

Much of an expert's knowledge can be transferred to a computer system. What is more, the computer system may then operate more rapidly and more consistently than the human

A heart pacemaker, electronic back-up for the heart's own sinus node. The microprocessor inside the pacemaker carefully times the tiny electric shocks sent directly to the heart muscle by a small battery.

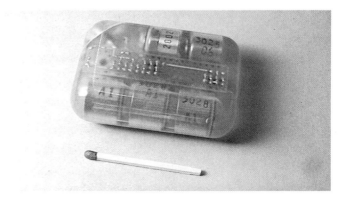

expert, at least within the narrow area of its expertise.

For some time it has been accepted that checkers and chess programs can play faster and more reliably than the human players who wrote them. It still seems alarming, though, to say the same thing about programs that make medical diagnoses. However, some of them consistently perform better than the consultants whose experience was used to compile their databases. Since databases are written in a way that prevents mistakes being repeated, their performance can continually be updated and improved.

Among the many successful medical systems in use are Puff, developed at Stanford University, California, which diagnoses diseases of the lungs, and Internist, designed at the University of Pittsburgh, Pennsylvania, which can analyze around 3 000 symptoms and diagnose about 500 different diseases. Other systems concentrate on advising doctors about drug dosages: Mycin, for example, deals with antibiotics. Other computer systems aid medicine in more mundane ways: for instance, by keeping track of medical records, or monitoring patients' heartbeats.

Another major area for research into expert systems has been geological prospecting. Prospector is a system which compares the characteristics of a geological area with models of different types of mineral deposit stored in its database, and then predicts the likelihood of finding particular minerals in the area. Dipmeter Advisor is more specific; it analyzes samples from a dipmeter, a device used in oil prospecting.

Computer-aided design

All these knowledge-based systems work by deductive reasoning, by drawing logical conclusions from the information made available to them. The computer excels in this deductive reasoning, but is less advanced in other forms of reasoning: induction, reasoning by analogy, creativity. Even so it can be extremely valuable to creative professionals such as architects, graphic designers and design engineers. Such people are seeing a massive change of job emphasis as the computer becomes an accepted design aid.

Computer graphics is a booming field. It is now commonplace for the computer to take co-ordinates in three dimensions and use them to construct a model on a video screen, rotate it in all three dimensions, overlay other details, change the scale and generally do all that a human designer can do on paper and more. Modelling systems used by engineers and architects can predict stresses, reject non-viable alternatives, and even suggest suitable materials and more efficient designs. The computer's ability to

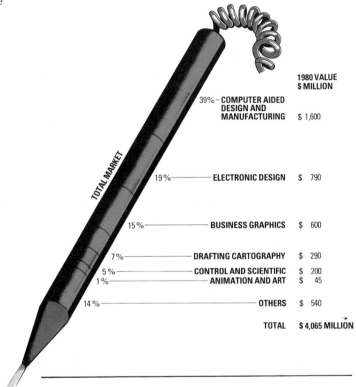

The relative importance of the various sectors of the computer graphics market (from Computerworld, UK, March 1981).

		1980 VALUE $ MILLION
39%	COMPUTER AIDED DESIGN AND MANUFACTURING	$ 1,600
19%	ELECTRONIC DESIGN	$ 790
15%	BUSINESS GRAPHICS	$ 600
7%	DRAFTING CARTOGRAPHY	$ 290
5%	CONTROL AND SCIENTIFIC	$ 200
1%	ANIMATION AND ART	$ 45
14%	OTHERS	$ 540
	TOTAL	$ 4,065 MILLION

TOTAL MARKET

generate an endless variety of alternatives at speed is challenging the human prerogative of ruminating at leisure over imaginative aspects of the design process. And the computer need not be restricted by built-in assumptions about size or shape which unconsciously lead human designers to rule out unconventional, but perfectly feasible, solutions to design problems.

One remarkable creative application in design is John, Julia and Peter Frazer's Intelligent Modelling at Ulster Polytechnic, Northern Ireland. The computer takes readings on the condition of a physical model from sensors and small microprocessors associated with building components. A designer, or a student, can interrogate the system about stress on structural members, heat flow from interior to exterior, maximum loading on different materials and so on. Plans, sections and perspectives can be computed, and the computer can display, enlarge and rotate all the images generated. Fed with specific requirements, such as a desired movement pattern for the inhabitants, Intelligent Modelling can propose structures that do not exist in the physical

Top right:
a Ford design engineer at work.

Bottom right:
computer-generated artwork. Given the original line image, the computer draws it to new scales and perspectives, rapidly and flawlessly.

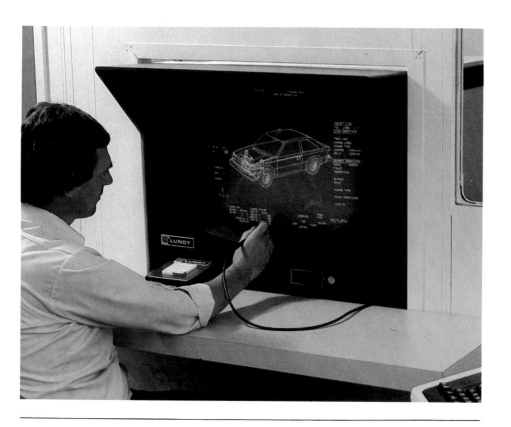

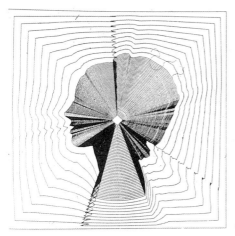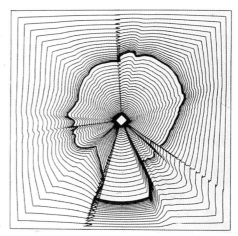

model, but that might plausibly be added to it.

Computer-aided design is becoming not merely useful, but indispensable, in another area: designing the complex components and systems that make up today's information environment. A computer can be programmed to design the complex integrated circuits that are eventually embodied in silicon chips. It translates the high-level symbols that define the various parts of the circuit into the lower-level wiring pattern that embodies the circuit logic.

Decision taking and decision making

The difference between two major categories of reasoning – deduction and analogy – is illustrated in the difference between two ways of using computers to help with decisions. Decision taking systems are deductive in style. Fed with data on past events, or personal preferences, they estimate the most probable or the most desirable alternative. All of them are based upon a particular method of taking chance and desirability into account (while statisticans dispute the foundations of both chance and desirability, there is little divergence over the methods used to take account of them).

Decision making is quite a different process. Here alternatives are not so much given as generated. The distinction is important when you are dealing with complex tasks like running a number of factories or commanding a fleet. For one thing, decision making under these circumstances involves learning, planning and inventing as you go along. Next, satisfactory estimates of chance or desirability are impossible. Finally, it is fairly clear that the ability to formulate a plan of action does not always go hand in hand with the ability to carry it out.

These points became clear in a series of conferences held by the United States Army Research Institute for the Behavioral and Social Sciences to look into the art of complex decision making. The conferences were small but selective; participants were authoritative, representative of different schools of thought. Traditional decision theories turned out to apply only to decision taking in the narrow, deductive sense. As the conference organizers (System Research, Gordon Pask's group) included more and more people who were not officially decision theorists, it became evident that a decision aid had to be much more than an aid to decision taking if it was to be effective.

Conference discussions stimulated research into a different type of decision aid, a sort of on-going model which System Research has since updated. This model was an evolving computer system called TDS or Team Decision System. The scenario has spacecraft protecting trade routes in space against marauders. A salient feature of TDS is that the space environment breaks apart if too much energy is expended destroying marauders in any one region, although it can be repaired by co-operative action. Any action (a simple instruction to a spacecraft or a sequence conditional on other events) becomes a tactic, which constitutes a program. The programming language consists of commands which control the spacecraft - the commander of a craft does not feel as if he or she is programming. Tactics are automatically translated into the Lp expressions discussed in Chapter 6, and they stand, in this form, as a knowledge structure.

Any commander is in control of at least two spacecraft, both autonomous, and both flying in space, the environment generated by a microprocessor. Co-operation between two or more spacecraft is real co-operation; both conflict and conflict resolution are genuine.

TDS can aid decision making by allowing the commander to interrogate the system; by giving information; by presenting the tactics currently in use; by doing calculations. But it also has an extra ingredient: there are real emergencies which parallel the unexpected emergencies of real life. For example, a spacecraft might run out of energy or be destroyed; trade might be irreparably disrupted; whole trading communities might perish; the space environment might become damaged beyond repair; navigation might become impossible; some or all of the trade routes might be destroyed...

However much the commanders interact with TDS as a decision making aid, they have no chance to deal with emergencies, simply because these happen too fast. In this case, they are given as much opportunity as possible to make decisions based on their own strategies and tactics. If there are five minutes or even five seconds left to make a choice, they can still select a strategy. But at 500 milliseconds there is no time for a human decision; TDS takes over and makes the choice on the basis of what it has learned about the strategies commanders have chosen in the past.

Interestingly, any one commander nearly always attributes this action to another commander, rather than to the TDS. In fact, it is all of them, machine and people, acting together.

The computer in research and development

TDS is itself a research aid as well as an aid to decision making. As behavioural scientists, System Research used it as a tool to investigate human methods of decision making. Some computer systems in education also have dual uses, as teaching aids and as research tools to investigate learning.

Computers act as aids in the physical sciences as well as the social sciences. Straightforward computation, the sorting of research data, and the modelling of complex systems all play their part in enabling scientists to do more work than ever before. And more subtle computer systems can help scientists to make, as well as take, decisions.

As a result, we are now seeing an explosion of successful research and development in all kinds of fields. One major field for such research and development is microelectronics itself. But increasingly, other fields – optics, biotechnology, neurology, cybernetics – are coming to interact with microelectronics, and to multiply its power. The boundaries between these fields of research are becoming blurred. The use of the computer in all these different areas is a co-ordinating factor, drawing out similarities in the knowledge structures used by researchers in each of them.

The co-ordination of these disparate technologies, and the tremendous pace of development in so many fields, are factors that are both quantitatively and qualitatively changing our perception of the world we live in. We see them as factors that are helping to bring about not only the information environment but also the emergence of the new species micro man.

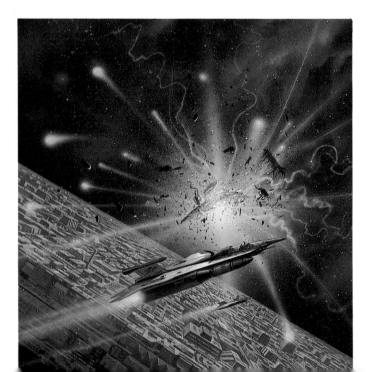

You are the commander of this space craft. You have 500 milliseconds to make a life or death decision. TDS, Team Decision System, takes over.

8 MAVERICK MACHINES

A computer that issues a rate demand for nil dollars and nil cents (and a notice to appear in court if you do not pay immediately) is not a maverick machine. It is a respectable and badly programmed computer. The time sharing system that wastes your time while you wait for its response is no maverick either. It is a computer suffering from overload, justifiable in the days when hardware was expensive but now simply irritating.

Mavericks are machines that embody theoretical principles or technical inventions which deviate from the mainstream of computer development, but are nevertheless of value. They have all worked at some stage and many of them are still working. Given an appropriate technology, all are potentially useful to the future development of computing.

They are also useful to our exploration of the nature of computing. They remind us that 'computer' does not necessarily mean 'silicon chip' – computing is possible using many other materials. They also demonstrate that the distinction between hardware (the machine) and software (the programs that run on it) is not as clear-cut as we may have made it seem.

Maverick fabric

You can make a computer out of almost anything. The London School of Economics once had an analog computer made of glass and filled with different coloured fluids that simulated national economies with a clarity that must have distressed mathematical economists. It used the same laws of hydraulics that operate the fountains at Tivoli just north of Rome.

There was also a generation of pneumatic computers. In these, switching was achieved by jets of air. This was serious technology in the 1960s and still has special applications, in reliable engine regulators, for example.

There have also been experiments using passivated iron (formed by the interaction of piano wire and nitric acid) as computing fabric, inert platinum electrodes as input and output devices, and zinc, light energy or electrical current as the stimulus to compute. Alternatively, computing structures can be 'grown' out of ferrous sulphate and sulphuric acid activated by electrical current; the resulting iron develops branching nodules known as dendrites, analogous to the branches of a program.

These two 'recipes' were combined by R. M. Stewart of California in 1963 to make a far more elaborate maverick device, essentially a resonant device with stable coherent cycles of activity. In place of piano wire he used steel spheres packed with

A hydraulic computer.

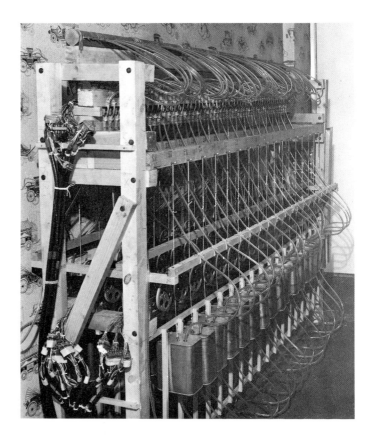

glass spheres, and silver or gold dendrites rather than iron. The whole contraption was enclosed in a container pressurized to 100 atmospheres.

There is no clear-cut distinction between the notion of programming (giving a system a set of instructions to be followed in a sequence determined by the outcome of operations included in them) and the notion of adaptation (allowing or encouraging the system to respond to the conditions it encounters). In the case of dendritic computers, where physical contact with the external environment is indeterminate, the two notions are particularly close. The simplest dendritic computers react to sound, vibration, electric light, and other stimuli, and therefore make no sense per se unless they are considered in the context of such stimuli.

By enclosing his arrangement in a pressurized chamber Stewart obtained more controlled effects. But the very ambiguity of the operations of devices like this has important implications. Because it is not easy to decide which components respond to vibration or which components compute the conditional reaction, the whole question of where the computer's boundaries lie becomes deeper and more complex.

There is now a demand for such devices, which are appropriate to non-logical forms of computation, but dendrites and regions of depassivation on passivated surfaces are physically too cumbersome for such demand to be met practically. It now seems that biological media may perform in similar fashion but on a more manageable scale.

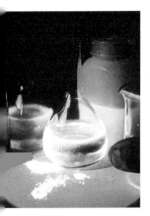

Chemical computing fabric?

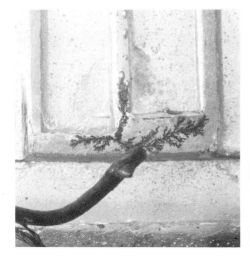

Dendrites growing inside a dendritic computer.

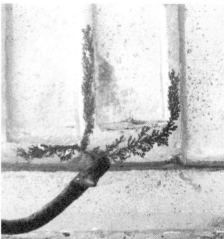

There are two important points to be made about non-standard systems of the kind we have just mentioned. First, different kinds of fabric may be peculiarly suited to certain functions. Second, fabric technology offers a great diversity of options only some of which are commonly developed. If the first proposition is accepted, more of these options ought to be developed for their appropriate purposes.

Millions of pounds and dollars, representing an incredibly large investment of thought and technology, have been expended in the manufacture of maverick machines. Often such machines have performed more effectively, especially in unconventional control situations, than standard operators. Maverick designs are quite well documented, but hidden away in conference proceedings or in the archives of funding agencies. One of the purposes of this book is to point out that this intellectual and monetary investment exists and that it should not be forgotten or squandered. People are, from time to time, apt to reinvent the wheel! And reinventions sometimes miss previous clever and crucial ideas, or stumble against obstacles which previous innovators succeeded in solving.

BOBCAT, a ballbearing computer.

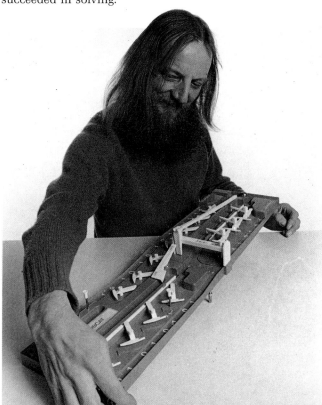

Mavericks
in control systems

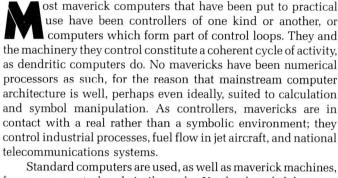

Most maverick computers that have been put to practical use have been controllers of one kind or another, or computers which form part of control loops. They and the machinery they control constitute a coherent cycle of activity, as dendritic computers do. No mavericks have been numerical processors as such, for the reason that mainstream computer architecture is well, perhaps even ideally, suited to calculation and symbol manipulation. As controllers, mavericks are in contact with a real rather than a symbolic environment; they control industrial processes, fuel flow in jet aircraft, and national telecommunications systems.

Standard computers are used, as well as maverick machines, for process control and similar tasks. Yet the thoughtful system designer is acutely aware of the difference between the symbolic environment of a program operating in a standard computer and the real world which it purports to regulate. The differences become obtrusive when the interface between the computer and its environment does not conform (and it seldom does conform) with the ideal of instruments to read and knobs to turn. Real reality is richer and more messy than that. It is much less in kilter with the internal symbolic world of a computer and its operating systems. Inevitably there are difficulties when one attempts to mesh the two worlds to form a coherent cycle of activity.

Standard computers owe their power to isolation. They are mechanical solipsists. Operating programs live in a symbolic environment consisting of the computer's binary code, its arithmetic/logic unit, and its theoretically infinite memory store. Within that symbolic domain, programs can weave patterns and structures which can be used to represent anything. But they are symbolic structures and it is we, ordinary people, who interpret them. With that interpretation – the attempt to fill the empty symbols the computer manipulates – the question of truth and falsehood enters the picture. Truth or falsehood is irrelevant within the symbolic world, provided the program's model of that world is a coherent one. The real issue is the truth or falsehood of the model in relation to the real-life situation it is applied to.

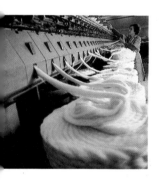

A wool factory – a real world to be regulated.

A system designer must specify, when planning a control system, the data it is possible to sample and the actions it is possible to take. In doing so, he or she has considerable freedom, including the freedom to allow for contingencies, such as overload, which have never occurred and maybe never will. At the same time, the situation to be controlled must be modelled in a form which the computer can manipulate. Here the designer comes up with a bump against the restrictions of the computer's symbolic world.

Perhaps the most important of these restrictions is one-dimensionality, the single perspective from which a conventionally programmed computer manipulates its data. The notion of counting and of serial ordering – the string-and-knot approach as we have called it – underpinned the development of conventional mathematics as well as computing. Only now are we beginning to free ourselves from this restriction. But the most powerful methods of escaping its clutches are not yet in common use in commercial and industrial applications of computing. Real environments do not usually satisfy the string-and-knot paradigm, a fact often overlooked because we unthinkingly describe and manage our environment using serial idioms. A vehicle assembly line, for example, is a serial idiom, although we seldom think of it as such.

How can we overcome this problem? One method would be to produce a model of the entire control system (the computer *and* the machinery to be controlled) which adequately represents the real system, and which can be computed on a serial basis. Another method would be to develop ways of manipulating more complex models inside a computer, or inside a population of computers. It is here that we re-enter, from a rather different direction, the domain of unconventional machines, maverick machines.

Unconventional programming

It is common practice for control systems to use data derived from the control process to modify the test and instruction values in their programs. All but the simplest feedback regulators do this. Computers commonly rewrite programs or generate new ones (an extension of the same principle) as a part of their control operations. In this way they adapt to changing circumstances, meshing the real and the symbolic world in the same coherent cycle of activity. However, there is an ordinance, commonly obeyed by programmers, that program construction shall not conflict or interfere with program execution.

Some programming methods allow the computer to carry out computations in parallel, in the sense in which microprocessors in nets and rings operate in parallel. But there is still a common controller, ensuring that the parallel operations never converge, that conflict never takes place. There may be several layers of programs, each adapting the program that forms the layer beneath it. But the model is strictly hierarchical, not heterarchical. It is more flexible than the original serial model, but not much so.

The black box

I t is not only individual acts of computation that are serially ordered. From a higher perspective, successive states of a control system suffer from the same limitation.

The computer-as-controller cannot be regarded as a physical black box, as isolated from the processes it controls. Rather it must be regarded as a functional black box, as having a boundary defined by an exhaustive specification of possible input data and output action, and as capable of assuming a sequence of successive, separate states. Any program or any selected program segment has to be evaluated before the result can be converted into an action upon the real environment. That action will then generate data which are input to the next program or program segment, and so on.

This sequence of calculation, evaluation, action and feedback is generally insisted upon as part of the logical process of controlling, in which it is assumed that the process being controlled can be distinguished from the controller, and must be evaluated by it. This limitation, though commonly observed, is not essential, and is in fact contravened in many maverick systems. As a result, the interaction between a maverick and its environment is far more complex than that between a conventional computer and the equipment it controls.

When a standard computer controls a real environment, it operates inside a fixed boundary of possible actions and possible data. The interface between the computer and its environment imposes seriality on its control transactions. A maverick machine, in contrast, is a piece of active fabric that computes and usually controls a real environment, but that works in a way which contravenes some or all of the limiting conditions normally imposed upon computers. It may, for example, fail to satisfy the string-and-knot requirement of serial processing; it may not evaluate the situation, or complete its calculation; or it may lack a fixed boundary.

Hybrid machines

A lthough there is an important theoretical distinction between analog and digital operations, in practice both can be combined. The result is a hybrid machine.

Most of the larger hybrid machines were built for special areas of application, such as controlling nuclear power plants or experiments in wind tunnels. At the time they were built, in the late 1950s and early 1960s, their hybrid nature was a matter of expediency; no other practical way of doing the job could be found. Today they would probably be replaced by digital systems combining many processors. However, the basic idea behind hybrid machines is still valid.

Hybrids store and execute a heuristic rather than a program. A heuristic can be defined as an open-ended series of instructions which are investigative and self-modifying; a heuristic proceeds according to trial and error rather than according to the fixed rules of a program. The instructions in a heuristic often call for concurrent operations of both the analog and the digital kind. In this context conflict can occur and so conflict resolution routines are included. This makes hybrid computers particularly useful in situations which do not even approximately fit the string-and-knot paradigm. They can control environments in which many partly independent processes go on at once, and where interaction between them may make it necessary to revise control instructions.

Modular machines

During the 1960s a much pursued avenue of research was the 'artificial neuron', or electronic module which imitated a brain cell. 'Bionics' was the general name given to these endeavours, which also included the investigation of other electronic devices with biological characteristics. Much excellent work on control and computation went on under this rubric. A modular machine is a machine that uses such computing elements.

Most modular machines operate on a 'threshold' logic, of which the simplest model is as follows. The module receives input signals in the form of electrical impulses. The impulses from several input connections are combined (in the simplest case they are summed or time-averaged) and if the sum or average exceeds the threshold value the module emits an impulse. Otherwise, it remains quiescent.

A heuristic process. The artist makes hundreds of tiny modifications and revisions as he draws.

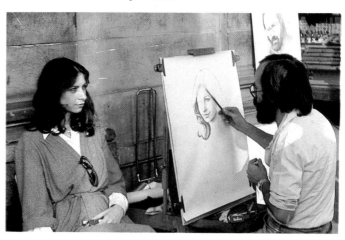

There have been numerous variations on this basic theme. Some modules emit trains of impulses rather than single impulses if their threshold value is exceeded; others emit longer or more frequent impulses depending on the extent of the excess. The threshold value may be altered locally; for example, if a module emits frequent impulses its threshold increases; if it remains inactive its threshold decreases.

The probabilistic state variable, or PSV module, is rather different. It consists of a small 'probabilistic' computer of the type pioneered by Roger Baron's group at Adaptronics, Washington D.C. Each module has its own random source of 'charge' that determines its state in relation to its threshold value. Its state is also determined by its input symbols, which can be thought of as adding a bias rather like the bias of a coin or a roulette wheel. From time to time the state of the module is assessed; if its threshold value is exceeded it emits an output signal. The assessment intervals may also be probabilistically determined.

There is a fundamental difference between a network of PVS modules and the operation of a computer system with a random component. In the latter the random number which resolves conflict between exclusive alternatives is just a further input, albeit 'stochastic' or arbitrary. In an asynchronous PSV network, the randomness applies not just to input, but to the system as a whole. The state of the system as a whole, not merely its input, is stochastically varied.

Modular machines are combinations of these modular elements, either several modules of the same kind or of different kinds linked together in a network that allows impulses to travel between them. The connections typically loop back, so that reverberatory cycles are often set up. The modules are capable of blocking the transmission of impulses to other modules, with the result that the network may functionally dismember into independent parts, temporarily or permanently. Seldom are all the modules active at the same time, and those which are inactive can at any time be recruited by functionally independent sets of modules.

Modular machines usually operate heuristically, their heuristic being embodied chiefly in the connections between the modules, which for special purpose applications are soldered, permanently linking the inputs of some to the outputs of others. Today, however, it is more common for these connections to be established by instructions from a microprocessor. In fact microprocessors can 'train' module networks to form suitable transmission patterns. Again, as in hybrid machines, there is no clear boundary between programming and adaptation.

All modular machines are effectively hybrid distributed processors. The computations they perform depend on the entire network of modules or on functionally independent sets of them. One design philosophy for distributed processors ordains synchronicity: all the modules must act together at specific master-clocked instants. However, asynchronicity has proved to be a more interesting and fruitful design philosophy.

In an asynchronous modular processor all the modules have independent clocks. This means that they act like the microprocessors in a network which does not have a common controller, or like a population of computers. The system self-organizes according to the signals exchanged between the modules. Typically regions of partial or completely synchronous activity develop as a result of the signals exchanged.

Among the first distributed modular hybrid machines were the Perceptrons of Frank Rosenblatt at Cornell University. These were designed to recognize patterns. Several single- or multiple-layer Perceptrons were constructed as synchronous devices. Later, asynchronous systems with similar structures were devised. These have a remarkable ability to control situations that do not fit the string-and-knot paradigm, situations that are liable to undergo sudden modification.

Such systems use their self-organizing abilities to replace any lost ability to control or compute should a module fail. An inactive module is simply recruited to play the same part as the failed module. In the sense that such networks use redundant modules to repair and reproduce functional units, and also to produce and accumulate new modes of computing and controlling, they can genuinely be said to learn.

It is intriguing to compare this form of computational redundancy with a rather strange property of the human central nervous system: the 'phantom limb' phenomenon. People who have had a limb amputated occasionally report being able to feel the limb, and the pain in it, as if the limb were still there. Sometimes it is possible to identify the nerve fibres responsible for the sensation and destroy them microsurgically. Logically one would expect this procedure to remove the 'phantom'. But in many cases the phantom returns. The sensation is the same but it involves other nerve fibres. In other words, the neuron activity which produces the sensation is transferrable. Neurons do not biologically replicate, so some form of computational redundancy must be involved. For some unfortunate individuals the nervous system seems to get better and better at reviving the phantom. No sooner are newly recruited neurons identified and destroyed than others take their place; destroy these and still

A real-life modular processor? Every element in this pond – weeds, algae, bacteria – is in some sense independent, but also controlled by day length, temperature and rainfall.

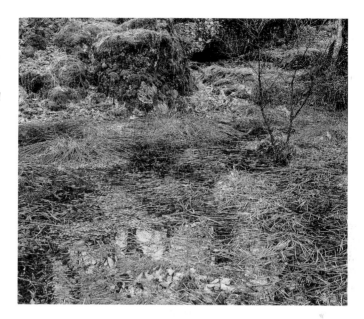

others take their place, with intervals between surgery becoming shorter and shorter.

In the 1960s and early 1970s the modules used in hybrid machines were literally bits of electronic circuitry you could hold in your hand, and they had to be wired together. Now microelectronics has reduced the size of both modules and connections to a scale at which they are not independently visible to the naked eye. One unit of visible size now accommodates many thousands of modules. The applications of modular hybrid technology are increasing, for instance in space vehicle control and satellite orientation.

Resonance and coherence

Let us go back a few years, and multiply component size several thousandfold. It is the mid-1950s, and I (Gordon Pask) had an interest in synaesthesia, the notion that there is a correspondence between musical forms, light, colour, movement and pattern. The idea had been around since the 1800s, and was especially popular in the 1920s.

It seemed to me and my colleagues that no absolute synaesthetic relationships existed, but that personal ones might be learned and used to enhance musical performance. Obviously, a device which did this would have to generate light patterns as well as learn about one or more performers. We constructed two machines which did this, and christened them Musicolour.

Musical input from a microphone was scanned by the machine's six variable filters, which were set up so that one looked for types of musical attack, two looked for rhythm and three for dominant pitch. The output from each filter went to a different adaptive threshold module, and the impulses from these determined the intensities of six banks of spotlights and the movement of associated light reflectors. The result was an interplay of colours and patterns.

Performers became addicted to Musicolour. By adjusting the filters it looked for variations on the status quo, that is on any original tune, rhythm, key and so on. The status quo was established by adjusting complex oscillators so that they resonated with the performers.

Musicolour was in effect the first coherence-based hybrid control computer. It worked by finding a method of coherence (a potentially loose form of knitting-together, as we saw in Chapter 5) that united the internal model of the machine with the external environment of the performers, and established a cycle of activity which passed from one to the other, and back again.

After using Musicolour, Chris Bailey of Solartron commissioned and part-designed a device called EUCRATES, after the sorcerer's apprentice. The first EUCRATES made its debut at the British Physical Society's exhibition of 1957, and was featured in *Time* magazine under the picture of a Jersey cow. But it had its serious side. About a dozen were marketed as special purpose hybrid computers, with a particular application as adaptive teaching machines. EUCRATES was the first coherence-based machine with a claim to respectability.

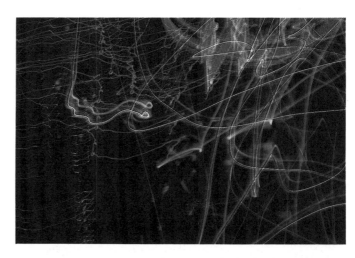

Light shows in night clubs and discos do not react to musical performers in the way that Musicolour did, by looking for and rewarding improvisation.

Simulation and reality

Though the design of the conventional computer imposes severe conceptual limitations, the computer *per se* is a flexible medium in which a wide variety of activities and situations can be modelled. The elaborate hierarchy of programs we have glimpsed, in which higher-level programs write or rewrite lower-level programs, is one instance of this power and flexibility. However, no matter how far the boundaries of the computer are pushed, conceptual limitations continue to reign in the world of the conventional computer. As a result, the models achievable must themselves be limited. In circumstances in which the inappropriateness of the serial paradigm becomes evident, the inappropriateness of the model constrained by the serial nature of conventional computing also becomes evident. In other circumstances, the model may adequately represent the truth of the real-world situation, but it is still a model, and not the situation itself.

Asynchronous modular networks may themselves be used as modelling media (for modelling neural activity for instance), but they are also a medium freed from the serial limitations we have discussed, a medium in which real activity takes place. If this activity is modelled in a conventional computer, the result is a model of the activity (whether the activity is itself seen as a model or not) flawed by limitations which do not exist in the real situation. Maverick machines offer a medium with capabilities that cannot be reproduced even by very elaborately programmed conventional computers, and they can be built from materials tailored to the computing processes to be carried out.

Do maverick fabrics have a future? Almost certainly they do,

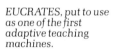

EUCRATES, put to use as one of the first adaptive teaching machines.

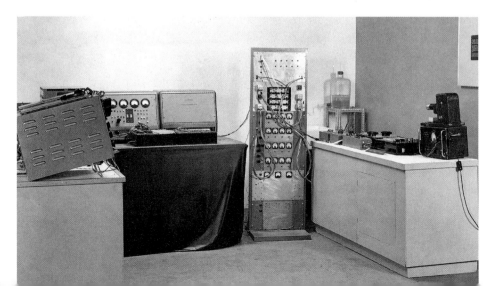

if they can be reduced to a size at which they become acceptable in modern computer technology, semiconductor or otherwise. As the fabric of computers gets smaller, the variety of physical effects which can be achieved tends to increase, although only a few of these effects have been exploited so far. At the same time the number of ways in which we can circumvent the limitations of conventional computing is also increasing.

The electronic technology of the 1960s, based on the thermionic valve, included about a hundred distinct sub-technologies. Today's microelectronic technology, based on the silicon chip, subsumes at least a thousand. The catalogues of semiconductor companies, with their strange acronyms, hint at the huge diversity of semiconductor and magnetic film media. Nevertheless, microelectronics does not rule the computer kingdom unchallenged. There is now a substantial technical base for optical computation, employing fibre optics and holographic effects in machines of small size and great reliability.

Another field that has grown rapidly but with few fanfares in the last 15 years is biotechnology, the deployment of controlled biological systems. The growth of biotechnology, and even its existence, has been made possible by computers. Conversely some of the products of biotechnology are fabric for computers, especially mavericks. Materials such as protein-lipid membranes, themselves the product of controlled biological processes, have switching, storage and oscillatory properties that offer new prospects for making systems self-organizing. Machines that are self-organizing on a biochemical basis may be better at modelling and controlling some real-life situations than conventional machines.

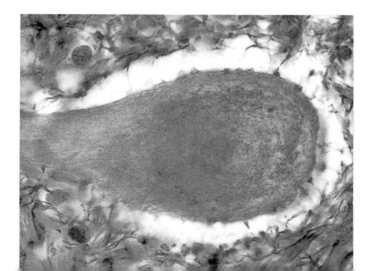

Other biological materials, and other properties of biotechnology in general, come more specifically into the area of semiconductors and conventional computing. But at this grain of detail, the borderline between living organism and machine becomes hazy. For example, is synaptic activity (the release and absorption of substances which carry electrical impulses across junctions between nerve cells and other tissues) a biochemical or a semiconductor phenomenon? The only honest answer to this question is both.

The term 'biochip', increasingly bandied about today, means different things to different researchers. For some a biochip is a single layer of protein molecules sandwiched between glass and metal, the individual molecules playing the same role as the silicon transistors of the conventional chip. Others see it as synonymous with chips made of conventional materials but possessing a complexity which approaches that of the human brain. Others see protein films and three-dimensional molecular assemblies as heralding a new era of miniaturization; already we have the technology to create chips containing 100 000 more 'switches' per unit area than conventional silicon chips.

Two biological switching mechanisms.

Left: a nerve ending or terminal bouton that transmits nerve impulses in one direction only.

Right: the layered structure of the retina. The pigments in the rod and cone cells (their nuclei show up as the thickest and darkest layer in this stained section) change their state according to light intensity. That change of state is signalled to cells in the optic nerve.

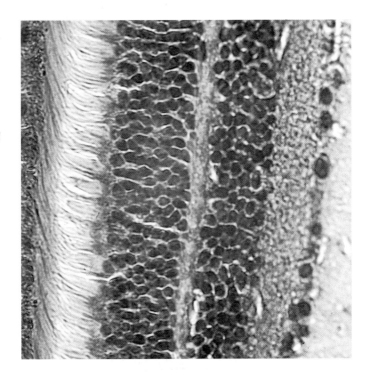

Chapter **9 THE PLUG-IN PEDAGOGUE**

'Where do we plug it in?'

It seemed a reasonable question, but the teaching-machine salesman looked puzzled. The year was 1960, the place a dusty suburb on the northern fringe of Los Angeles. California hadn't quite left for the twenty-first century, but it was preparing for lift-off. Gordon and 'the English lady travelling with him', to quote from a slightly puritanical report of the period, had come to California for a glimpse of the future.

After a moment, the man nodded towards a wall socket. We plugged the machine in and switched it on. Its screen showed a picture of an apple, a pear and a concertina, along with the cryptic message: THE APPLE IS A, B OR C?

The salesman seemed perlexed, even offended, by the lack of an immediate response on our part.

'Could an apple be a B do you think?' Gordon wondered aloud.

'It could, I suppose' replied his companion. *'After all, 2 x 4 can be "multiplication" as well as 8'.*

The salesman remained silent. Gordon pressed button B and kept it pressed. The machine presented, in rapid sequence, pictures of various fruits before halting, unexpectedly, on a banana. There was a smell of hot insulation. A wrapped candy emitted from the backside of the instrument fell to the ground. There was an embarrassed pause.

'A reinforcer?' we asked. *'You know, for getting it right?'*

The salesman gave us a hard look.

'Yeah, a negative one.'

He breathed in and became not quite a salesman-psychologist.

The incident really happened. Not all 'teaching machines' of that era were as stupid as that one. But some of them were. Later, at a party, we met our salesman again. After a few drinks he forgot that he'd seen us before.

'Hey' he said. 'You could plug it in here' and pointed to his cranium. 'See, the brain's a teaching program, right? It's optimal, tested, right? All your behavioural objectives wired in, right?'

'No, wrong...'

'It's one daddy of a great idea, though...'

Was it? Stuffing knowledge into a vacant head, as grain is stuffed down the throat of a Strasbourg goose? Is knowledge like grain or mind like the belly of a goose? Anyhow, what is the equivalent of *pâté de foie gras* as the end product? We had, and have, serious doubts about the whole endeavour.

Machines, computers in particular, acquired a rather tawdry image in educational circles because excessive claims were made for them and little was actually achieved. With hindsight it

Computerized teaching was anticipated long before the computer came along! This nineteenth-century French cartoon imagined school life in the year 2000.

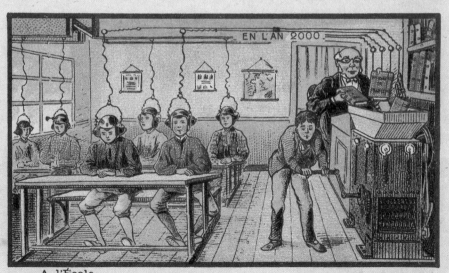

EN L'AN 2000

A l'École.

would have been better public relations to forget the term 'teaching machine' and use 'instructional device' (for academic-type learning) and 'training aid' (for skill learning) instead. The comment is poignant today, for it is not the machines as such which are important, but rather the methods of learning, instructing or training used. The relevance of the micro is that it has made a wider range of methods practical, even possible.

The educators who are currently exploring how computers can be used to impart skills and knowledge are in the vanguard of research into how learning takes place. What is more, attempts to teach computers human skills like language are teaching us how to use computers to teach humans more effectively.

Early adaptive instructional machines

One day in 1957 Norman Crowder and I (Gordon Pask) encountered each other over a cup of coffee and SAKI, my adaptive keyboard instructor. Norman said that he too had invented an adaptive machine which, like SAKI, increased the difficulty of the tasks it set the student as the student's proficiency increased. He delved into his pocket and brought out a programmed textbook (with pages to be looked up in a sequence depending upon the response to questions posed) which was something of a disappointment. 'It's as good as my machine', he said, a very honest remark from a man recognized as a pioneer in the field of computer-aided instruction.

Norman Crowder's machine, like many that came later, was indisputably memorable: a horrendous whirring contraption, built to last, which fast-wound and fast-stopped rolls of cine film containing reams of instructional, descriptive or remedial material. The electronics which linked all this gadgetry to the student's console functioned as a rather complex computer. Being a general-purpose instructional aid the machine had to be reprogrammed as well as reloaded for each course. Depending on the student's answers to questions and his or her past performance, the machine's program would branch adaptively, opening up harder and faster, or easier and slower, routes through its material – very impressive and sophisticated.

Norman was underplaying his machine. It is true that the principles used by his machine and its program are the same as those that could be used in an impracticably elaborate programmed learning text where students have to estimate their level of proficiency, use a table to determine where to turn next, and then search for the appropriate material. But the machine has a charisma which no programmed book can have, and it did behind-the-scenes work that would have fully occupied, and infuriated, a student.

The good machines of the 1960s (Crowder's machine was one example of that class) were just as good as an individually dedicated computer, and in those days were far less expensive. They did not sell as well as they should have done partly because computer phobia made people hesitant to try them, and partly because this kind of instruction, the presentation of set bodies of material, has limited applications. Also (and this was the point Crowder made by handing over the programmed textbook) no machine can be better than its instructional program, and the manufacture of good programs is a skilled and costly job. At any rate, it was never possible to develop a sufficient variety of programs to give these early machines a wide market and so reduce the hardware cost. As a result, machines like these never became a generally available resource.

Skill training

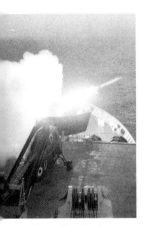

Firing a Sea Dart missile, which is computer controlled. These missiles proved their accuracy in the Falklands conflict in 1982.

Progress in the field of skill training – imparting not only facts but also the ability to perform specific tasks – was not as difficult as progress in the field of pure instruction. Although none of the machines we know of were great commercial success, because the markets for them were very specialized, a number were commercially viable. Devices which catalyze and speed up the acquisition of critical skills are usually one-offs and very expensive, but nevertheless cost-effective. Performance requirements are easier to specify for skills such as fault detection or parts assembly than in academic fields. Also the process of learning a specific skill fits better into the psychological model of learning and reinforcement on which the machines and their programs were based. Felix Kipstein, Ernst Rothkopf and Larry Biggs in the United States, and Max Sime, Bernard Dodds and Harry Kay in Britain were among the many researchers who were active in the 1960s in the field of computer-aided skill learning.

Obviously a training machine must give the student something to do, monitor his or her performance, and use data derived from that performance to modify the training program and tell both student and supervisor how much progress is being made. The more interesting training devices are both adaptive and predictive. An adaptive training machine contains a model of the task in question, and an outline model of how the task may be learned. As the program accumulates information about the student's progress it fills in its outline model with the details. Equipped with this information and the specifications of the task in hand it will then predict which sub-tasks the student will find easy or difficult. It will then present sub-tasks of a suitable level of difficulty, and check its predictions against the student's

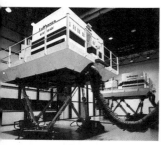

One of the most advanced uses of computer modelling is in flight simulators used to train pilots. This Rediffusion Boeing 737 flight simulator is used by Lufthansa at their training centre in Frankfurt.

Computer management of training

The computer is not a replacement for the teacher; the microcomputer (right) is only a teaching tool like the coloured cylinders (far right), but more sophisticated. The teacher's human touch is needed in both cases.

performance. It modifies its activity so that the student's performance is maintained at some predetermined level, or, in more interesting systems, at a level which is modified during the learning process.

Experience with such machines showed that the best results came from accurately matching difficulty against performance so that students never became bored by a succession of easy tasks or overwhelmed by a succession of incomprehensibly difficult ones. During the 1960s Gordon Pask's group employed a general purpose hybrid trainer in the laboratory and also designed practical skill trainers for many different purposes.

Flexible and adaptable as such systems were, it was necessary to dedicate a machine to one student at a time, even though it could refer to a large computer for information or problem-solving aid. Dedication was an expensive undertaking in the pre-microprocessor era, and the application of such systems was limited as a result.

Computers can also be used in less capital-intensive ways to enhance the training of skills. In computer-managed scheduling, for example, the computer acts as a general resource allocator to the training program, handling the efficient allocation of trainees, equipment and human instructors. Another approach is computer-managed instruction, in which the computer controls the overall task sequencing of each trainee, though without actually guiding the trainee through the performance of each task.

The computer can also provide a database of information about the skill being learned, and can be interrogated when a student gets into difficulties. A very successful system of this kind has operated for years as an assembly line trainer at Hughes Aircraft in the United States. After some briefing about the product and the background of the job, apprentices are placed directly on an assembly line and do quite complicated operations, usually stages in the manufacture of electronic equipment. This is possible because they receive detailed visual and graphic instruction from a computer-like output terminal. The terminal tells them about the components in front of them, how they are put together, and what to do if something goes wrong. This is literally on-the-job learning. Eventually the computer's help becomes unnecessary, but if an individual gets into difficulties, he can recall the training program. Trainees are issued with their personal computer identity card on which the computer writes details of their training schedule and the progress they are making.

Computer-managed instruction in schools

Similar methods can be applied in schools and colleges. The Hatfield computer-managed instruction mathematics program in Britain was initiated by Bill Tag and his colleagues in 1970. It covers the entire school district, and the computer (the Hatfield Council's own central processor) plays an essential, but deliberately minimal, part in its operation.

Mathematics workbooks and answer sheets are issued and used in class. Copies of the students' completed answer sheets are collected by van every few days, coded, and centrally processed in one batch. Programmed instruction is built into the printed materials, so that scoring and more subtle evaluation is possible; so are remedial exercises for students who have failed to grasp a point. But these materials are not the sole means of instruction. The system complements direct tuition by the teacher; the processed data allow the teacher to pinpoint the needs of individual pupils and provide them with the particular support they need.

One essential feature of this scheme is the periodic updating of course materials. Another feature of paramount importance is that teachers are implicated at all levels (from curriculum to graphic layout) alongside the computer team, both in creating and updating the system. It is possible to produce a very detailed learning history for each child over the year and to revise teaching schedules accordingly.

Education

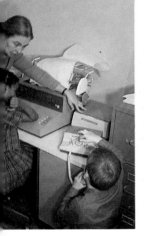

Methods used to teach practical tasks can also be applied to the teaching of academic subjects such as history or geography. However, there is a qualitative leap to be made between imparting data (facts linked in a relatively arbitrary way) and imparting bodies of knowledge. The application of computers to academic learning began with the former

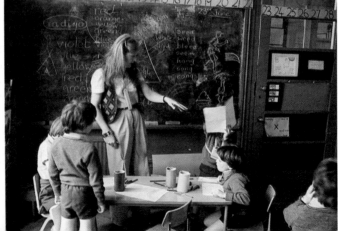

and has now moved on to the latter. The very rich and complex discipline which has emerged is known as educational technology (sometimes applied epistemology) and it embraces learning, educational psychology, computer systems and knowledge structures.

The first general applications of computers to academic learning were utterly banal, little better than the candy-spewing machine with which we opened this chapter. The early systems performed simple branching operations and reacted (on the whole, slowly) to answers which could have been given more conveniently by filling in boxes on a multiple-choice question paper. The inadequacy of these early systems was partly due to delays caused by time-sharing across too many terminals. Even so, some excellent mainframe systems did and still do exist. A more fundamental problem was the odd conviction – on the part of systems designers with a naive and over-simplified view of educational psychology – that the word computer, intoned religiously, would miraculously solve all teaching problems.

It was hardly surprising that teachers were often offended. It was fortunate that the behaviouristically oriented psychologists at whom the twaddle about computerized teaching was chiefly directed were cautious about machines as serious aids to education. American behavioural psychologist B.F. Skinner experimented with teaching machines, but he regarded them as a demonstration, not as a basic tool. Susan Mayer Markle, an expert on programmed learning based in Chicago, had a very sceptical attitude to computers as a vehicle for learning.

Some computer-based educational systems with a single centralized processor serving many terminals can be effective if properly employed. Nevertheless it is the smaller, inexpensive, dedicated microprocessor that is beginning to have a revolutionary impact on education. Some of the earlier unfortunate experiences may have delayed this impact, but they have not prevented it.

SOCRATES

SOCRATES – the acronym for Systems for Organizing Content to Review and Teach Educational Subjects – was probably the first serious attempt to use a single central processor to control a dozen or more student stations. It was designed between 1961 and 1963 by Lawrence Stolhuron of the University of Illinois and it achieved, as intended, a Socratic or question-and-answer dialogue with each student. It could refer to a central library if necessary and could also call in a live teacher if the tutorial rules proved inadequate for a particular learning difficulty.

Although SOCRATES was limited by the response format, it closely resembled some of the best centrally controlled systems in use today in that it posed and solved problems in ways that encouraged real student involvement and innovative thought.

PLATO

PLATO is an interactive computer system designed primarily for computer-aided instruction (the acronym stands for Programmed Logic for Automated Teaching Operations). Its uniqueness resides partly in its hardware set-up and partly in its enormous range of software options.

Don Bitzer invented PLATO in 1960. By 1961 it was operating on the Urbana campus of the University of Illinois. At that time there were some 25 terminals in one large room, together with a complicated electromechanical device rather like an oversize juke box that selected slide graphics. It had excellent display facilities and proved to be a great success.

The PLATO learning system has spread widely since then. There are now more than 60 learning centres in North America and a number in Europe as well. Each centre has a number of dedicated terminals linked to a mainframe PLATO computer. Private terminals can be linked to the system as well. At Illinois the emphasis is on demonstrative instructional programs. The term 'demonstrative' is applied to programs that provide simulations that allow students to discover results which are often not intuitively obvious. One of these is a biology program concerning the reproduction of fruit flies, where the student gives the genetic make-up and the computer shows typical progeny. Another offers a smog map of Chicago: the user gives the system a wind direction and the computer produces a pollution overlay. Now that Control Data have taken over the system on a commercial

One of the useful aspects of teaching with the PLATO scheme is that multiple-use terminals are provided. Each of these people is conducting a separate dialogue with the PLATO program.

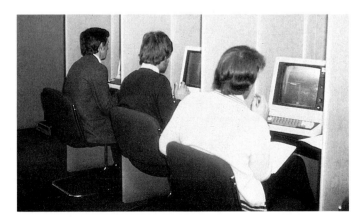

basis, its emphasis has changed to business-oriented programs. In London, for instance, the programs offered include 'EXCEL: Professional Excellence in Your Job', and 'Selling: The Psychological Approach'.

There are negative aspects of PLATO. For example, its mainframe time-shared basis means slow access on any but underloaded systems. There is joke among users that when someone comes for a demonstration all they get is the PLATO spiral, a signal indicating that the system is at work; and when they do get the program menu the best lessons are often unobtainable. This is not quite fair, but there is more than a grain of truth in it. However, considering the early date at which its fundamentals were laid down, the PLATO concept has worn exceptionally well.

TICCIT

Victor Bunderson and Bob Merill at Brigham Young University, Utah, adopted a Mitre Corporation computer-controlled colour cable-television system as the basis for their work. Their TICCIT system minimizes the shortcomings of centralized computing. Its main advantages, apart from its colour video display and local data storage system, are a thoughtfully worked out relational data structure (an educationally tuned form of the relational databases mentioned in Chapter 6) and a clear authoring language which provides examples and counter-examples of topics and topic definitions. A TICCIT microcomputer system with enhanced demonstrative capability is now becoming available.

Interactive learning

Both PLATO and TICCIT depend on the lesson concept, a lesson being a batch of programmed material which students absorb at their own pace. However, this is only one mode of using computers in education. Increasingly computers are being used interactively, as tools which enable people to learn by doing. They do not provide knowledge in the form of lessons, but act as catalysts for the acquisition of knowledge.

An example of interactive instruction in geography is shown below. This particular program encourages children to find out for themselves what the most important factors are in choosing a site for a village in the year AD 600.

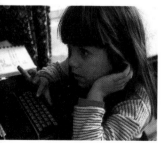

It is amazing how fast young children are at mastering a micro-computer keyboard – the necessary preliminary to 'talking' with the machine.

I HOPE YOU HAVE THE MAP OF THE AREA IN FRONT OF YOU. WHERE HAVE YOU DECIDED TO ESTABLISH YOUR VILLAGE? TYPE IN YOUR CHOICE NOW AS IN THE EXAMPLE. (EG. A/2)
← C/3

Choosing a site for a village. Interactive programs encourage students to explore alternatives and discover why some are better than others.

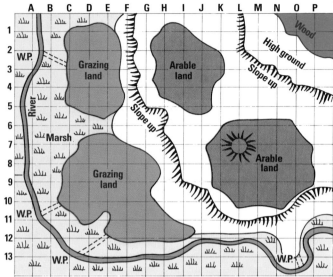

W.P. = Water-point – can only be reached by track. = = = = =

THIS SITE HAS AN EFFICIENCY RATING OF 35.
NOTE. THE LOWER THE EFFICIENCY RATING, THE BETTER THE SITE.
THE RANGE IS BETWEEN 1 AND 100.
TRY TO CHOOSE A BETTER POSITION.
TYPE IN YOUR NEW CHOICE NOW.
← N/10

THIS SITE HAS AN EFFICIENCY RATING OF 43.

CLEARLY SOME SITES ARE BETTER THAN OTHERS. LIKE YOU EARLY SETTLERS WOULD HAVE NO WAY OF KNOWING WHICH WAS THE BEST POSSIBLE SITE. THEY WOULD HAVE MADE A RATIONAL-SENSIBLE CHOICE BUT ONE CAN IMAGINE THAT A GOOD DEAL OF TRIAL AND ERROR WOULD HAVE BEEN INVOLVED. TURN TO PAGE 2 OF YOUR BOOKLET AND READ WHAT IT SAYS THERE.

WHEN YOU ARE READY TYPE CON TO CONTINUE.
← CON

NOW TRY TO CHOOSE A BETTER SITE FOR YOUR VILLAGE.
TYPE IN YOUR CHOICE NOW.
← N/12

THE SITE HAS AN EFFICIENCY RATING OF 37.

THERE NOW FOLLOWS A DESCRIPTION OF HOW THE COMPUTER WORKED OUT THE EFFICIENCY RATING FOR THE LAST SITE.

DISTANCE FROM VILLAGE TO RESOURCE AND BACK AGAIN

NUMBER OF VISITS IN A TWO WEEK PERIOD

WATER 38MMx30=1140MM
GRAZING 80MMx15=1200MM
ARABLE 44MMx10=440MM
FUEL 184MMx7=1288MM
BUILDING MATERIAL 184MMx2=368MM
TOTAL 4436 (EFF.RAT.37)

IT MEASURES THE DISTANCES IN MILLIMETRES (MM) ON THE MAP FROM THE POINT CHOSEN TO THE NEAREST POINT OF EACH RESOURCE AND THEN DOUBLES THESE DISTANCES TO ALLOW FOR THE RETURN JOURNEY. IT THEN MULTIPLIES THE NEW DISTANCES BY THE NUMBER OF VISITS IN EACH CASE. IT CONSIDERS ONLY THE NEAREST WATER, GRAZING LAND, ETC. IT THEN ADDS UP THESE DISTANCES TO OBTAIN A TOTAL. THE TOTAL IS THEN CONVERTED INTO AN EFFICIENCY RATING FOR SIMPLICITY.

IF YOU FOLLOW THIS PROCEDURE WITH A NUMBER OF SITES YOU WILL BE ABLE TO WORK OUT WHICH WILL INVOLVE THE LEAST WALKING DISTANCE. THE SHORTER THE DISTANCE, THE BETTER THE POSITION.

NOW IMAGINE THAT YOU ARE HAVING TO ESTABLISH YOUR VILLAGE IN TROUBLED TIMES. YOU MUST CONSIDER THE PROBLEM OF DEFENCE. WHERE WOULD YOU SITE YOUR VILLAGE NOW?

TYPE IN YOUR CHOICE.
← 0/9

THE DEFENCE RATING IS 90.
AGAIN THE LOWER THE RATING THE BETTER THE POSITION.

THE RANGE IS AGAIN BETWEEN 1 AND 100.

THE EFFICIENCY RATING IS 47.

YOU MAY NOW HAVE FOUR FURTHER ATTEMPTS TO
IMPROVE THE DEFENCE RATING OR TO FIND AN
EQUALLY GOOD POSITION. REMEMBER YOU WANT TO
KEEP THE EFFICIENCY RATING AS LOW AS POSSIBLE
STILL.
WHERE WOULD YOU SITE YOUR VILLAGE NOW?
TYPE IN YOUR CHOICE.
← C/3

THE DEFENCE RATING IS 20.
THE EFFICIENCY RATING IS 35.

One of the most innovative uses of an on-line computer is
Arie Dirkzwager's project at the Free University of Amsterdam. A
fairly small machine is networked out to high school terminals;
these can be used for individual study, but also in a class setting.
A student, or a small group of students, tries to solve mathematical problems at the terminal, but the display is made visible to
the entire class on a large television screen. The problem-solving
process provokes lively debate, with the teacher making comments and the students trying different solutions at the terminal.

Computers are particularly well suited to demonstrative
uses. At the University of Naples, for example, there is a
simulation that allows students to determine a sequence of
isothermal, adiabatic and isobaric operations on a gas, and to
discover that certain cycles of operation eventually bring the gas
back to its initial state.

Similar techniques, making full use of the colour graphics
now available on many microcomputers, make computers useful
as tools for teaching very young children. Special simplified
touchpads and joysticks, instead of the full alpha-numeric
keyboard, enable even three-year-olds to communicate with the
computer.

Advanced Learning Technology, a company set up by a
group of educationalists and programmers in 1979, concentrates
on producing educational programs aimed at young children.
These use colour graphics and sometimes synchronized tape-
recorded speech and music. They run on the Apple range of
microcomputers, and include a set of imaginative games with
letters and numbers which feature Bumble, a cartoon creature
from another planet. Another ALT set of programs, Juggler

Skills, is aimed at three- to six-year-olds. These use graphics to teach concepts such as above and below, left and right, and encourage children to match sound to picture.

Children a little older than this tend to move on from using ready-made programs to writing their own programs. Already, many competitions have been set up to encourage junior programming. One precocious offering was a computer dating program that matched up every male with one female, and vice versa, to ensure a no-conflict Saturday night (the inventor of this was Donald Abrams of New York). Another offering was a stock analysis system by 17-year-old Matthew Korn, also from New York. Other schoolchildren have developed an analog-digital musical synthesizer, speech synthesis programs, and even a program that predicts the spread of fires.

LOGO, an educational language

High-technology can be fun! Below: an array of the electronic learning games now being marketed for small children. Centre: a LOGO turtle – it moves according to simple programs that children can easily create for themselves, and draws pictures with its central pen. Right: turtle controller at work.

arly in the 1970s Wally Feurtzig and Seymour Papert of the Massachusetts Institute of Technology developed a programming language, LOGO, specially for use by youngsters, though adults enjoy it too. Papert has been pursuing the educational impact of LOGO over the years, improving it and extending it. His studies are careful and tailored to individual learners, mostly in schools. Papert was a colleague of Jean Piaget, the famous Swiss child psychologist, and his work has a depth and a realism seldom found in work based purely on controlled laboratory studies or on massive survey data.

Today LOGO is used in computer installations in the United Kingdom (at Jim Howe's organization in Edinburgh, for example) and also in many places in the United States, and is now becoming available as a microprocessor facility. Its emphasis is on discovery, on learning by doing, and it has a flexibility

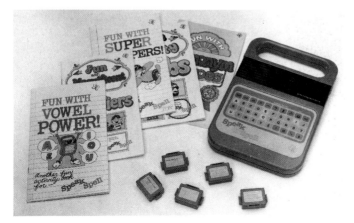
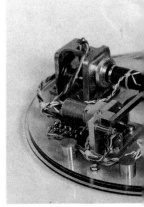

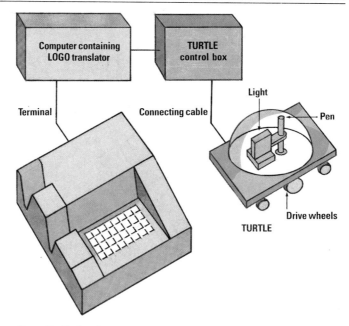

Computer containing LOGO translator

TURTLE control box

Terminal

Connecting cable

Light

Pen

Drive wheels

TURTLE

Typewriter Keyboard

LOGO programs are typed in on a terminal keyboard; the computer translates them into a sequence of commands; then the control box transmits the commands to the turtle.

and simplicity which allows users to engage in a wide range of operations from mathematics to music. A particularly interesting option is Computer Geometry. A LOGO program drives a 'turtle' – either a picture that moves around on a video screen or a simple robot controlled by the computer. In either case the turtle can be made to move various distances in various directions, drawing lines on the video screen or on a sheet of paper. Terminals and turtles can be assigned to one individual or to a small group.

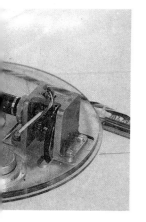

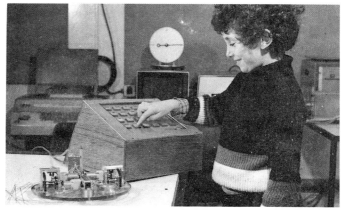

LOGO is useful for learning simple programming, but it goes farther than this. As children learn how to program they also learn to understand their own thought processes. Tuition, assistance, suggestions and discussions may be initiated by a teacher, or by the students themselves. Whether used to follow a syllabus or to encourage group learning and participation, LOGO has proved an excellent tool for innovation and discovery. It has even been used successfully by artificial intelligence researcher Sylvia Weir of Edinburgh University as a way of getting autistic children to relate more openly to the world around them.

These then are some of the many computer programs that act as dynamic and demonstrative instruments in education. Nearly all design aids, decision aids, traffic simulations and process simulations can be used in education, and many of them have been, very successfully. Increasingly, the teaching of skills appropriate to a specific job is being merged with education proper. Take suites of planning programs, for instance. One program might accept statements about all the facilities required in a building and produce a bubble structure of all the ways in which a specified area might be filled with them. Another program in the suite, if given critical dimensions, might generate floor plans. Another, given additional data, might generate the outlines of what a building containing all those facilities arranged in a certain manner would look like. Is this a design tool or an educational tool, or both?

Probably the richest computer environment in the world is at the Washington D.C. Children's Museum. It is based on a complex of computers, peripheral devices and a stock of software which offers the chance of writing programs as well as using them. Are the people who go to the Museum being educated? There is no clear-cut answer to this. But of one thing we can be quite sure: computers are steadily changing the face of education.

Knowledge representation in schools

A major advantage of computers is that they can indicate what topics are to be learned, how they are connected together, and (having picked up information about your style of learning) how you might learn them most expeditiously. In the context of LOGO the necessary overview is provided by a real-life teacher who asks questions such as 'Why did you model the situation like that?'

Any education system must have some kind of knowledge structure. The question is, what kind? We are plagued by preconceptions about learning that stem from thinking that schooling is synonymous with education. Few people deny that the Children's Museum is educational in an exploratory, creative way. But a museum is not a school.

As an institutional necessity most schools have periods, classes, examinations, curricula and syllabi. Certain topics are supposed to be taught in particular settings and at particular times. These institutional requirements echo the hierarchical concept of knowledge; they are the outward expression of the well worn notion that easy topics should be learned first and difficult ones later.

But there is no good evidence that learning in general proceeds in this way, even if teaching sometimes does. It would be absurd to depict the exploratory learning that goes on at the Children's Museum, for instance, as a hierarchical process. It is equally absurd to imagine that all children, or all adults, find the same topics easy or difficult.

All the same, learning in schools is likely to go on in this way for some time – the hierarchical model becomes a self-fulfilling prophecy. This does not mean that computer-aided instruction systems should be hierarchically structured, although sadly most of the early systems were. We are not seeking to deny the importance of schools. We respect them as places where youngsters learn to get on with their peers and with adults, and where they learn to accept and profit from a measure of supervision, discipline and guidance. Formal teaching has many advantages, but learning under such a system is never as efficient as exploratory learning. No two children learn the same, even when they are part of the same group or helping each other on the

Fears are often expressed that our machine society will turn us all into apathetic cogs in some grand mindless mechanism. These boys learning computer programming look very unapathetic: vigorous interest shows in every face.

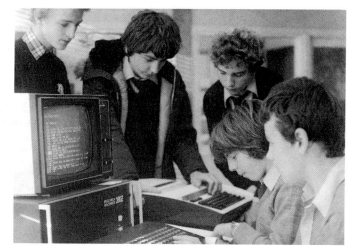

same project. And almost certainly both of them will learn differently in different contexts.

There is no intrinsic reason why educational computers should be used to further formal teaching methods. In fact there is every reason why they should not, because they are especially good at handling non-hierarchical knowledge structures. By their versatility computer programs can promote analogical reasoning, invention and creativity as well as deduction and simple inductive inference and their structures are capable of evolving as new topics are understood.

Just as training can open out into education, so education, at its best, can open out into discovery and the creation of new ideas and designs. Schooling, in the sense of training rather than social learning, is a small part of education.

Educational possibilities

Over a period of 11 years (five of overlapping projects and a six-year research project) the Social Science Research Council in Britain supported a study by System Research (Gordon Pask's group) on learning and knowledge. The group collaborated with other researchers in England, Europe and Canada who were working to develop effective methods of teaching statistics, physical chemistry, biology, history, physics, psychology and genetics.

The results of this research, some done in the laboratory (simulating real-life conditions) and some in schools and colleges, revealed many educational possibilities and also a number of obstacles.

Below: nothing could be more 'mechanized' than old-style school teaching. This 1816 watercolour shows a classroom in Harrow School, Britain's most famous public school.

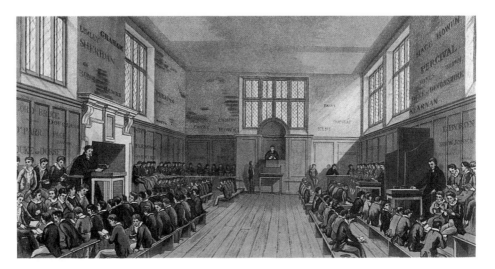

One of System Research's basic tools was a computer-regulated interface, CASTE (Course Assembly System and Tutorial Environment). With CASTE, people did not talk *to* the computer, but *through* it. CASTE was designed chiefly as a means of making people act out the concept-building process, usually a hidden mental process. At the same time it provided answers to such questions as How do people teach themselves? and How do they teach each other when they are in groups?

The principle underlying CASTE was the conviction that understanding is achieved by saying how something is done, doing it, and saying why you did it in the way you did.

In the System Research work, we started out with the idea of a knowledge map, accessible from many points. It turned out that this approach, though less restricted than the linear model of a classroom lecture or a textbook, was still too restrictive. Given this much liberty people wanted more, and gained by having more; the computer had to be programmed so that their knowledge maps evolved. This also proved too restrictive. So the calculus of the protologic Lp described in Chapter 6 was programmed. Under these circumstances CASTE operated as follows: students selected one or several topics; then they were presented with a selection of relevant learning strategies; then they chose the strategy that most appealed to them.

People adopted an amazing diversity of learning strategies — often analogical, sometimes step-by-step, sometimes global. The patterns that finally emerged were largely due to the influence of school training. Style is a property of a person in context, not of a

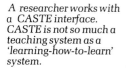

A researcher works with a CASTE interface. CASTE is not so much a teaching system as a 'learning-how-to-learn' system.

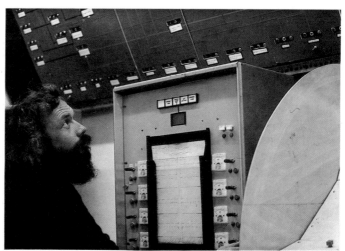

person alone. We found, however, that at an individual level people had their own characteristic approach to learning. The important lesson here was that if teaching strategies are mismatched to students, no relevant learning takes place.

Two other important lessons were learned, both from work in the laboratory and in schools (where transportable versions of CASTE were installed). No matter what the subject matter, a strictly applied CASTE routine, requiring full understanding at each stage, was superior to classroom or textbook instruction. However, by reducing the rigour of CASTE students could be given the experience of what it means to understand rather than having systematic understanding of each topic forced upon them. One surprising finding was that less stringent CASTE was more effective after an incubation period than stringent CASTE; information was retained better and problem-solving became more innovative. Students 'learned to learn' and, in particular, to create analogical relationships which aided understanding. Having learned to learn students used personal manoeuvres to continue the process and no longer needed the computer except, occasionally, as a means of modelling.

The main negative conclusion was that timetables and fixed classroom periods make it difficult to implement effective learning strategies in a school context. Human understanding cannot be conveniently squeezed into fixed time intervals.

Until recently there was no practical way of overcoming this difficulty inexpensively enough to make a strong impact. Wellintentioned encouragement of analogical reasoning within an old institutional context is not enough. But there are now ways of making computer-aided learning far more efficient and costeffective. It is now feasible to provide computer facilities for individual students, enabling them to schedule their own learning. Networked facilities with access to a knowledge structure (such as Lp's Thoughtsticker) stored in a large central computer can free teachers for individual teaching. They can also keep a record of each student's progress.

Micros in schools today

The age of microcomputers in schools - and in homes, for education takes place there too - is with us. Commodore Business Machines (Pet series micros) and their user group held the first Pet Education conference in London in 1981.

Even in the present austere economic climate, grants are being given for microprocessors in schools. In Britain and the United States, and elsewhere in the industrialized world, most schools will soon have at least one microcomputer.

The other essential ingredients, namely staff and student

acceptance, are present and growing too. Nick Rushby of the CEDAR project, based at Imperial College, London, tours the United Kingdom demonstrating micro-type ideas and sounding attitudes. The BBC's Computer Literacy Project, launched in February 1982, received 50 000 enquiries before its first program was shown on television, and many of the microcomputers built to BBC specifications and marketed by them are going to schools. Similar developments are taking place in Canada, Sweden, Belgium, Holland, France and Italy. It is the recent development of amazingly cheap and easily available microprocessors that is leading this metamorphosis of education.

But that is not the end of it. Anne Floyd and Tim O'Shea, using ingenious micro-based equipment developed at the United Kingdom's Open University, are studying people's styles and learning strategies with ten or more times the efficiency that System Research was able to achieve. Ranulph Glanville at Portsmouth Polytechnic and other British colleagues are using microprocessor networks to aid and influence approaches to a wide range of design problems. They have demonstrated that knowledge acquired through actually designing something is qualitatively different from knowledge gathered from textbooks. At the Architectural Association in London, for example, most learning is design. This kind of learning goes on all the time as a natural function of the way we understand the world. Perhaps microprocessor-based systems will become prosthetic aids to the human mind, amplifying the natural learning process and demolishing artificial barriers to knowledge and understanding.

Perhaps the man at that party in Los Angeles had a point when he suggested plugging the pedagogue into his cranium. But the pedagogue (if that is what our mental prosthetic is to be called) will not stuff facts into our skulls. Instead it will catalyze the aesthetic of exploration, the delight of knowing, and the joy of creating and sharing concepts.

Chapter **10 THE INFORMATION ENVIRONMENT**

In 1973 a telephone 'pirate' was prosecuted for manufacturing a 'blue box'. This device was particularly popular in Boston, Massachusetts. It enabled the user to make telephone calls around the world for no more than the few pence an ordinary

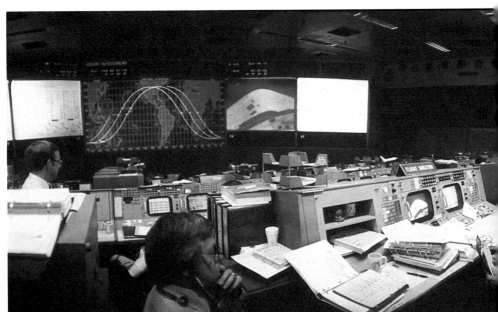

local call costs; it worked by sending a sequence of sound tones into the telephone, giving the user access to the international switching network. It is rumoured that the first 'pirate' to subvert the computers that route international calls used a plastic whistle found in a box of breakfast cereal.

Underlying this apparently trivial anecdote is a point of great significance: were it not for the fact that large switching networks of this kind are now entirely computer-regulated, a fraud of this sort would not have been possible.

The world we live in today contains large numbers of computerized communication and control systems that are becoming less and less separate from one another. National and international systems are being linked to form highly complex information networks. These networks constitute what we call 'the information environment'. Indeed the information environment can itself be thought of as one vast distributed computer.

A major theme of this book has been the idea that linking computers together in ways that introduce the possibility of conflict, and of conflict resolution, will lead to greater complexity of computer thought and application. Nevertheless all the systems mentioned in the first half of this chapter are expressly designed to avoid the possibility of conflict. They do not conform to our definition of a population of computers; they are merely

International communications networks are so complex that it would be impossible to co-ordinate them without computers. The same is true of special-purpose networks, such as satellite tracking and command systems. Below left: mission control at NASA in Houston, Texas. Below right: a radar tracking installation at Mount Longont, Kenya.

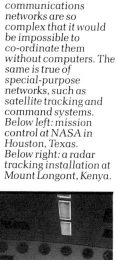

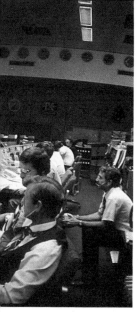

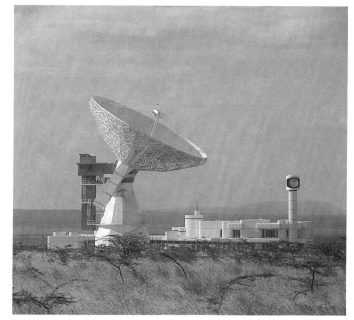

networks of computers. Nor does the information environment of which these systems are presently part constitute a population of computers. Populations of computers are perfectly compatible with an information environment but they do not, even margi- nally, exist in the information environment of today.

Even so, the present information environment is bringing about major attitude changes. These have little to do with the far more radical revision of thought that will take place when comfortable distinctions between human thought processes and machine thought processes become blurred. These changes are essentially quantitative, brought about by the daily, massive increase in powerful computing capacity.

Let us look first at some of the constituent systems of the present information environment and then explore some of the consequences of linking them together.

Information systems in buildings

Were the elevator controls, humidity, temperature and energy controls, intruder alarms, intercoms and security systems of any large department store built before World War I looked on as information systems? Probably not, but they were just that. Were the overhead pneumatic tubes and wire tracks used to communicate with a central accounts office seen as communication networks? Probably not, but they were just that.

Information systems in buildings are nothing new; they existed before computers were even thought of. The real heart of an information system is the way in which computation, communications and control enhance each other and magnify the capability of the system as a whole. Control need not even be centralized. All the same, most modern information systems are designed around one or more microprocessors which provide both centralized control and computational capability.

A good example of a building control scheme was that set up by Motorola Semiconductors in 1979 in a demonstration house in Arizona. The system was co-ordinated by five microcomp- uters. The occupier of the house communicates with the system via a standard television set, which acts as a video display unit, and a keyboard. Originally, the system was set up to control the temperature and heating of the house and to run a security system but it could equally well have been extended with a computer games facility or a message sending and receiving centre. The most obvious advantage of domestic systems like this is energy saving. Lighting and heating can be kept at levels which maximize both economy and comfort. Unfortunately the low insulation and building standards of many houses render such systems less effective than they might be.

Domestic systems like this can incorporate a variety of alarm systems, programmed to sense everything from burglars to fires. They simulate occupancy when the house is empty, switch lights on and off and even play snatches of pre-recorded dialogue. Their various sensors might even be linked to the video display unit of a local security company or to the local police and fire stations.

The West Canada headquarters of Gulf Canada Limited in Calgary is one of the most energy-efficient large buildings in the world thanks to its computer-based control system. Eight hundred sensors throughout the building analyze environmental requirements and feed data back to the computer that controls the highly efficient and economical heat exchange system. Another computer controls the building's elevators, monitoring traffic and matching elevator journeys to user requirements. There are obvious analogies between this system and systems used to control road traffic.

A business information system: the London Stock Exchange

The London Stock Exchange is a typical specialized information system. Information is the essential commodity of the Exchange and has been since its inception, but today that information is manipulated by computer.

The Exchange is a clearing house for price quotations, company news, commodity news and news of more general economic and political significance. Some of this information is retained in house or on networks to which access is controlled. Some is sent to clients – other private networks, news agencies, and the media. Information is routed to and from the main computer via some 25 input and 25 output points in house. The system's database contains around 30 000 pages of information, and a wide variety of programs manipulates this data to provide collations, forecasts and statistics. Each day around 10 000 changes are fed into the database.

The system is also linked to a viewdata-type system called TOPIC and to a cable television system. At least 1 000 microprocessors are associated with the main processor, but they are distributed around various terminals, and printing devices.

At both the business and technological level, the London Stock Exchange has intimate links with other stock exchanges around the world. Transactions in London depend on transactions on other stock exchanges working different hours, and the London database has to be updated with information from these other exchanges. The entire system forms a kind of international game, where the players in London begin at 9.30 am, five hours

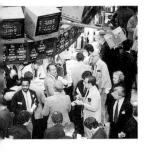

Brisk dealing on the London Stock Exchange. Over 1 000 microprocessors orchestrate this apparent turmoil.

earlier than in Wall Street, and retire at 5.30 pm, nine hours later than Tokyo. But where is the umpire? Who controls the system, at the business or the technological level? We no longer know.

Point of sale systems

The kind of information required by retail stores concerns customer purchases, stocking, re-ordering, profit margins, fast- and slow-selling lines, customer credit ratings and so on. In a typical computerized point-of-sale system today, a wide range of information about each purchase is fed into the system by an enhanced electronic till. Many supermarkets make use of bar codes marked on all merchandise. A bar code does not actually contain the price of the item – this is fixed centrally and can be changed without re-marking each item – but when that item is purchased the bar-coded data are read into the system via an optical wand or light pen, the processor identifies the item from its bar code, and the till flashes up the price. Full details of the item are reproduced on the customer's till receipt, and the same details are used by the central processor for the purpose of re-ordering and producing sales statistics.

Point-of-sale terminals can also be used to check customer credit ratings. The internal information system of any store is potentially linkable to a huge information environment consisting of the databases of many different stores, credit companies, hire purchase companies, banks, manufacturers, service companies... Eventually it will be impossible to say where one system ends and another begins, just as it is already impossible to make sense of transactions on the London Stock Exchange without reference to stock transactions elsewhere in the world.

This W.H. Smith book warehouse at Swindon in the West of England is almost empty of people, yet it maintains a stock of over 24 000 items and distributes them to hundreds of retail branches all over Britain. Stocking and despatch are controlled from the terminal room below.

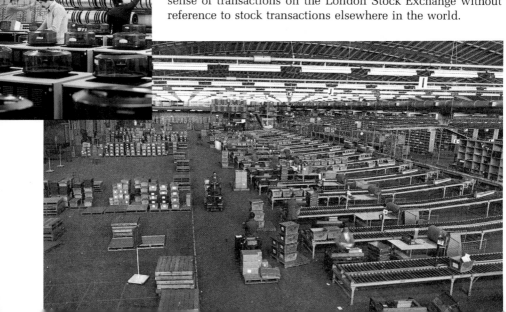

Electronic transfer of funds

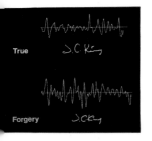

True   ∂.C.K⌐

Forgery   ∂.CK⌐

Linking retail stores with credit card companies is one example of the electronic transfer of funds. In Britain the first link of this kind was between the Army and Navy Stores in London and the American Express British Centre in Brighton, itself linked by satellite to the American Express data centre in Phoenix, Arizona. No real money or paper records are exchanged, only electronic coded signals. In time such systems can be expected to coalesce into a much more universal scheme for transferring money electronically, networking together many thousands of financial institutions and retailers. Progress so far has been rather slow because of the fearsome security aspects of such systems.

Telecommunications

Telecommunications lie at the heart of the information environment. They are by far the most common means of linking processors and the other components of information systems together.

In the early days of the telephone system, the impulses generated when a number was dialled triggered electromechanical relays in the telephone exchange, and these determined how calls were routed. As the number of telephone lines grew, however, this method of routing became impractical. Eventually large numbers of small computers were introduced to perform the operations necessary between dialling and routing. Tommy Flowers, mentioned in Chapter 1 in connection with the Colossus code-breaking machines, was one of the pioneers of this system in Britain.

In the United States the situation was slightly different. To make the operations of the giant Bell system compatible with those of smaller corporations, it became necessary, at a very early stage, to introduce large mainframe centralized computers and digital peripheral devices.

In the early stages telephone speech was transmitted in analog form. Today, however, converting speech into digital form has distinct advantages. For example, analog signals degrade over long distances but digital ones can be boosted en route. System X, now used in Britain, is a digital system. It is of modular construction, allowing exchanges to be adapted to fit growing numbers of subscribers and types of service.

The simplest device used to interface speech and other sounds with digital codes is the 'modem' or modulator-demodulator: this converts analog sound signals into digital code and vice versa. More elaborate devices are needed for viewdata systems, which transmit graphics and text. The trend today is to provide each telephone subscriber with 80 000

Above: signatures on cheques can now be verified by computer scanning.
Below: the heart of British Telecom's telecommunications system: the top of the Post Office Tower, a highly visible structure, once the object of terrorist bombing, rising high above central London.

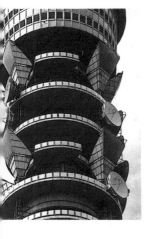

bytes/second of line capacity (an expression of the rate at which signals of any kind can be transmitted). This is sufficient for speech, colour graphics, telex and most computer connections. Much higher rates of data transmission are available for special uses. In nearly all cases the equipment linked through a distributed exchange system contains one or many microprocessors. The telephone itself is still the exception, but soon it too will be controlled by a microprocessor.

Many of the lines that connect telephones to exchanges and to computing systems are still conventional copper cable, but increasingly copper cable is being replaced by fibre optic cables, coaxial cables and microwave links.

Today the switching functions of telephone exchanges are combined with the computing and control requirements of the telephone company via exchange processors. These not only route calls but also keep accounts and carry out statistical and reliability checks. They do lots of other jobs as well, such as identifying the type of data being transmitted and decoding or interpreting it, determining the type of channel available, monitoring traffic flow, and creating and retaining files of programs. The close meshing of computation, communication and control functions achieved by exchange processors has dissolved the barrier that once existed between computers and exchange equipment. Computers, or rather exchange processors, are the equipment.

Satellite links

Very high frequency radio waves behave like light beams. They can be focused and reflected from suitable antennae, and can then be beamed in a particular direction to impinge upon, say, a satellite in orbit. This is the method of communication used by satellite links. The satellite is fitted with transducers that receive messages transmitted in digitally coded form via radio waves and then retransmit them, using a lower frequency, to a different point on the ground.

A number of types of satellite link are currently in use. The simplest is designed for rapid transmission of data from one fixed point to another. Europe's biggest nuclear physics laboratory, CERN, in Switzerland, for example, has a satellite link with Britain which can transmit information at the rate of 100 megabytes/second.

Satellites also form part of more complex communication systems linking many transmitters and receivers in a satellite version of the ring systems discussed in Chapter 3. A satellite ring might link the computers in a town, a large laboratory or even a large industry.

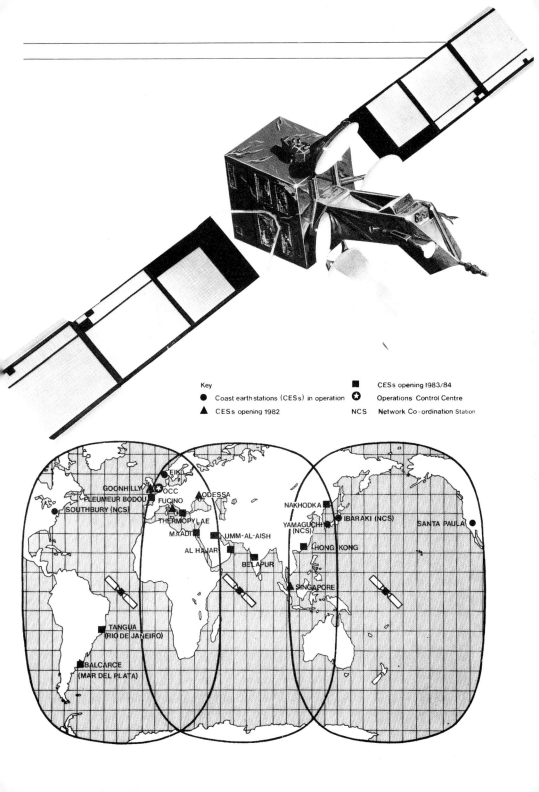

Key

● Coast earth stations (CESs) in operation

▲ CESs opening 1982

■ CESs opening 1983/84

✪ Operations Control Centre

NCS Network Co-ordination Station

EIK

GOONHILLY

OCC

PLEUMEUR BODOU

FUCINO

SOUTHBURY (NCS)

ODESSA

THERMOPYLAE

MAADI

UMM-AL-AISH

AL HAJAR

BELAPUR

NAKHODKA

YAMAGUCHI (NCS)

IBARAKI (NCS)

HONG KONG

SANTA PAULA

SINGAPORE

TANGUA (RIO DE JANEIRO)

BALCARCE (MAR DEL PLATA)

The satellite-systems revolution (from T.R. Ide, The Computer and the Communications Revolution, *workshop paper for the Club of Rome, February, 1981).*

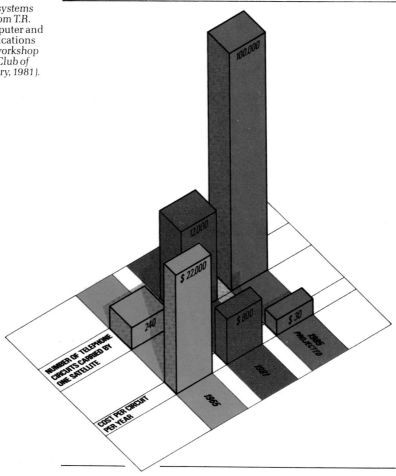

The emerging information environment

Terrestrial networks of telephone and telegraph operations work under different priority and cost constraints from satellite operations. Other areas of the information network – the postal system or the air transport system for instance – may be in competition with them or serve slightly different markets. Defence and diplomatic systems form yet another layer of computation and communication, linking in to the rest of the information environment.

The burgeoning information environment however is not only the product of increasingly cheap and powerful microelectronic hardware combined with the bringing together of hitherto distinct information systems. It is also a product of the interac-

Below: 'biotechnology' is all the buzz today, but we have been using some of the life forms used in biotechnology for thousands of years ... in the brewing industry. There's more to beer than you think!

Bottom: a holographic plate showing the keys of the city of St. Petersburg (now Leningrad). When lasers are sent through the plate a three-dimensional image is formed, apparently hovering in space.

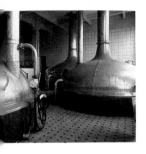

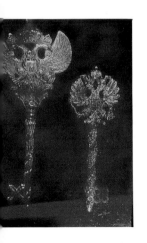

tion between distinct technologies. To put it at its simplest, microelectronic technology has multiplied our knowledge and use of other technologies. The most important of these in computing terms are biotechnology and optoelectronics.

Biotechnology, as mentioned previously, is the industrial deployment of natural and semisynthetic agents of a cellular or microcellular kind. These agents are used in all manner of industrial processes. Biotechnology emerged partly as the result of increasing refinement of familiar processes such as brewing and wine fermentation, and partly as the result of laboratory techniques developed for genetic engineering research. Redesigned using products such as structured protein-lipid membranes, any of the maverick machines we described in Chapter 8, which at the time seemed evolutionary dead-ends, could become very much alive.

Biotechnology represents the possibility of control at the smallest possible physical scale. Its products are serious competitors (perhaps partners) with the semiconductors of conventional microelectronics. Dr. James McAlear, head of the biotechnology company EMV Associates in Maryland, predicts that by 1983 his company will be producing test versions of a biological microchip, working in three dimensions, which provides 100 000 times the capacity of any of today's silicon chips. The microscopic circuit designs will be deposited, in gold, silver or lead, on a protein chip, and the protein will then organize and rearrange the non-protein, as in living organisms, to provide a vast number of molecular switches.

Optoelectronics is the generic term for a number of technologies that combine electronic control with conventional optical technology. Among them are fibre optics, the technology that produces cheap, efficient cables for transmitting digital signals in the form of light flashes, and the technologies that produce the liquid crystal displays and light-emitting diodes one sees in digital watches. A major field in optoelectronic research at the moment is flat screen television; Japanese firms working in this area hope to put thinned down large-screen television sets on the market by 1984. Flat screen prototypes use a variation of the liquid crystal technology used in digital clocks.

Another aspect of optoelectronics is holography, the production of three-dimensional photographic images. Holographic media may well become viable for the storage of large amounts of data in computer-readable form. Holography has already been used not only as an art form, but for marketing displays, making records of three-dimensional objects, and for a security card system, Data Card International's Access Control System.

The role of cybernetics

Another major factor in the pattern of development of the information environment is the application of cybernetics (the general theory of systems, including but not limited to communication, control and computation systems) in integrating psychosocial and physical-biological processes. The hyphen in this last adjective is deliberate, since the distinction between living and non-living processes is at present indistinct, both in theory and practice. Many psychosocial adjustments must go hand in hand with the physical-biological growth of the information environment. Perhaps the most important adjustment (discussed allegorically in the next chapter) is in the meaning we attach to the terms 'service industry' and 'employment'.

From evolution to revolution

The information environment is with us now. All the major technological developments that underpin it have already taken place. The number of networks in existence is more than sufficient to justify the term 'information environment'. The linking of networks, and the merging of technologies, is a reality.

What we have been describing in this book is a process of evolution on a number of fronts. Technical developments are often exciting and in recent years they have been particularly rapid, but it is difficult to point to any date which can be taken as a watershed, as Day One of a revolution. We cannot state with conviction: 'This and this and this were discovered in 1970 and they changed our world'.

Where is the revolution then? Where revolutions always occur: in people's minds. In other words, it is not the technology we possess that is so vital but the way in which we think of it and the use we make of it.

Cultures and the technologies that support them – not just information technology but transport technology, industrial technology, military technology, agricultural technology, and all the rest of the technological infrastructure – are real because some combination of thoughts, processes, beliefs and styles of life make sense together. They are coherent rather than incoherent; connected rather than disjointed; synergistic rather than interfering. There is conflict, but there are also means of resolving it. Once an organizational system is established it reproduces itself, quite literally, in many different ways. Novel methods of maintaining the system are developed, making it productive as well as reproductive. As a rule, novel entities which arise within the system (inventions, advances in technology, new philosophies of life) will be coherent with it. If they are not, the social pressures that sustain the system will either reject or pervert them.

The use of semiconductor technology is a good illustration of the inbuilt conservatism of culture. There are many potential uses of silicon chips; some of them have been put into practice, some are under development, and some have never even been contemplated. The prevailing tendency has been to use them to develop machines in the image of small computers. Other uses have lagged far behind. Why? We believe it is because the inbuilt conservatism characteristic of any culture rejects those uses which might upset the status quo. Creating small computers poses few dangers. Creating an integrated information environment poses many more. Creating some of the environments outlined in Chapter 11 (all of them based on technologies we possess today) is revolutionary.

There will always be theories and inventions that remain unexploited, that never get off the ground. There are others that exist as small research projects, or movements with a clique of faithful adherents, over many years. But the less orthodox interactions that go on between small organizations usually pay deference to the larger interactions that form the cultural norm. There is a tendency for smaller schools of thought, or political theories, or research programs, to be assimilated into the mainstream, occasioning only minor adjustments in the status quo. This is not revolution but conservative evolution; the organization simply accretes more means for achieving the same ends. It becomes stable by virtue of redundancy, and as it ages and becomes entrenched the pressure to do the same sorts of things increases. New technologies and theories, initially destabilizing, become stabilizing.

How then does radical transformation ever take place within a culture or an organization? Rarely is the majority of a population enthusiastic about changes of a kind which could be described as revolutionary. One has only to think of the reception given to automation, except of the most limited and mass-production-oriented kind; in Britain and in many other countries it has been, at the most, lukewarm.

We believe the answer lies in the fact that as a productive and reproductive organization ages, and becomes stable by a redundancy of means for achieving the same ends, so also it becomes more vulnerable to external influences of a kind that may or may not be deliberately disruptive. The assimilation of a novel idea, technology or industrial process (some novelties must be accepted to sustain the evolution of the organization) becomes increasingly likely to produce either an altogether different organization, or a fundamental split. The French mathematician René Thom calls this occurrence a 'catastrophe'.

In this context, the word does not necessarily mean 'disaster'. To put it succinctly, if at an advanced stage of entrenchment any norm is modified, it becomes increasingly likely that a revolution will occur, and that the existing norms will change as a result.

Employment in the information sector

We are seeing the emergence of a new culture. Our old culture is that of an industrial era; our new culture is that of an information era. And we are starting to adopt the lifestyle, the technology and the ideas appropriate to an information era, perhaps without realizing it.

The changing importance of what have until now been thought of as the three major sectors of employment is shown in the graph opposite. Here we come up against a difficulty: the framework used for classifying employment in an industrial society is not entirely appropriate in an information society. Our

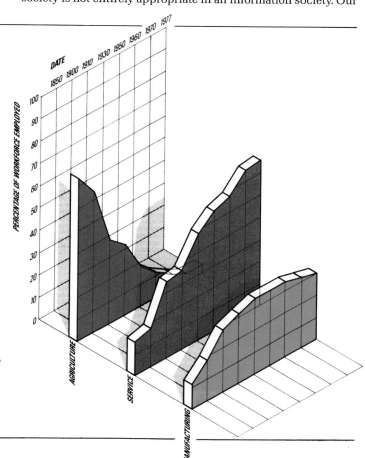

Employment patterns in the United States from 1820 to 1977. The agriculture and service sectors have virtually swopped places (from Encyclopaedia Britannica and ILO Yearbook of Labour Statistics).

idea of what we mean by 'employment', and how it is related to concepts such as 'work' and 'pay' is changing. So, too, is the way in which we classify jobs into different categories – agricultural, manufacturing, service, and so on.

The statistic of most interest to us is the percentage of workers engaged in information handling – people working in office technology industries, people using the products of office technology (computers, word processors, telephones, telex machines), people in the media, and so on. This statistic is not easily extractable from the familiar statistics that divide us into agricultural, manufacturing and service workers. Obviously our new category of information handlers would include many workers previously classified as service workers, but also many workers included in the manufacturing category (information handlers working within manufacturing organizations).

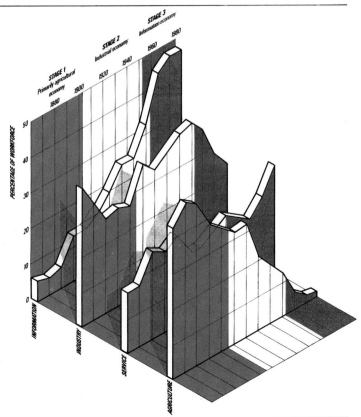

The changing structure of the United States work force, 1860-1980. Stage 1 was predominantly agricultural and Stage 2 predominantly industrial. Stage 3 is the world today, mainly and increasingly an information and service economy (adapted from R. Curnow and S. Curran, The Silicon Factor, 1979).

In practice, virtually all jobs involve some information handling; far fewer consist of nothing but information handling. It is clear that the number of workers within the information sector is growing rapidly, as shown in the last graph. A recent survey estimated that 46 per cent of the United States work force handled information, and that in the next decade this figure is likely to rise to 60 per cent.

Predicting future patterns

Can these trends be extrapolated into the future? In some dimensions it seems likely that they can. In others they may prove deceptive as pointers.

Clearly there are national differences in patterns of commercial exploitation and of research and development. In Britain the limiting factor is usually commercial exploitation, whether that involves developing a full-scale prototype or implementing full-scale production. For example, the British Post Office's System X exchange system, which is being installed throughout the 1980s, is based on a system that was operating as a pilot in 1968. Even today, its electromechanical predecessors are still being installed. In contrast, the limiting factor in the United States is usually research and development rather than commercial exploitation. This leads to different patterns of research and economic activity.

Once a technology exists, it can be exported piecemeal to other areas where comparable circumstances prevail, for example to other countries with similar infrastructures. Will the emergence of the information society reinforce existing inequalities between nations, confirming the currently rich and poor as the informationally rich and poor? Or will it bring about a narrowing of the gap between developed and developing countries, as the less developed take advantage of technology?

Countries that import technical knowhow, at any stage from blueprint to finished product, abolish part of the time lag involved in the development cycle. In the modern world it is relatively easy to import the sort of knowledge that underpins the information environment, and most developed and developing countries are actively doing so. The imposition of an information environment, however, demands the existence of an infrastructure, both physical (an efficient electrical grid, for instance) and mental (an educated work force). It also demands investment capital. It is upon the creation of this infrastructure that most developing countries are concentrating their resources.

A developing country has little to gain today by introducing a significant industrial phase before moving over to an information society. True, the industrial phase is the period in which a country is supposed to generate its own productive capability in order to reduce its dependence on imported goods; but unless an industrial phase is considered desirable for strategic reasons, it is economically more sensible for a developing country to import foreign manufactured goods, and to concentrate on nurturing an information environment. The high technology industries of the information environment are just as capable of earning foreign revenue as heavy industries such as steel refining.

A serious recipient of transferred technology will generally opt for the most advanced technology available. When this technology is applied in an entirely new area, rather than in an old one, another time lag, created by the obligation to live with viable but obsolescent systems until they can be written off or brought up to date, is abolished. Similarly the main practical

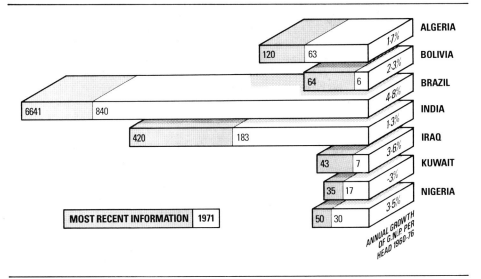

Increase in the number of computers in developing countries (adapted from Juan Rada, The Impact of Microelectronics, ILO, 1980).

limitation on incorporating microelectronic control into, say, electromechanical postal or telephone networks is the need to maintain compatibility with existing equipment, so that services are not disrupted. But for countries without large-scale existing networks, compatibility is relatively unimportant.

All these considerations mean that a country such as China, where there has been a determined effort to enter the advanced information-based stage of development, can move rapidly from a position of virtually no computing capability to the acquisition of a growing capability based on machines several generations in advance of those in use in the West.

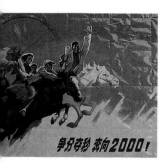

The future is rushing towards us, even if we are not rushing towards it. This poster from the Chinese People's Republic exhorts everyone to 'Take advantage of every minute and second to race to the year 2000'.

The difficulties caused by a dearth of national resources are often overestimated. It must be borne in mind that industrialization in the information era is far less costly in real terms than it was in earlier eras. However, many commentators, among them Juan Rada of the International Labor Organization (*The Impact of Microelectronics*, 1981), feel that on balance a combination of positive and negative factors could work to increase rather than decrease existing differences between nations.

Certainly there is little sign as yet of a technology ceiling at which the advanced nations will stick while the developing countries catch up with them. It is generally accepted that microprocessors and memory storage devices will continue to become more powerful, more compact and cheaper throughout the rest of this century, and probably at much the same rate as in the past 20 years, although there is always the possibility that microelectronics may further increase the pace of research and development.

Has the revolution already occurred then? Or is an even greater revolution still ahead of us?

In Europe and the United States computer-mediated developments have reached a point at which we believe they are irreversible. But these developments are not yet complete, partly because many people retain attitudes and ways of thinking born of the Industrial Revolution. It is when these attitudes change to match the new patterns of technology and work that we shall really begin to appreciate the extent of the changes taking place, and they will be comparable in their overall social impact with the invention of numbers or of the printing press.

In the rest of the world, development is at a less advanced stage. It may not even take the same course. Indeed, social and cultural differences will probably ensure that it does not. But we believe that by AD 2000 most of the world will be living in an information society of some kind.

Directing the changes

Cultural preferences will play a major part in determining how the future information environment will be shaped. We believe it can be shaped, as we show in the next two chapters. But that fact should not blind us to another qualitative change which the information environment has brought about. Even today it is an environment containing processes which, in a literal and physical sense, cause it to reproduce and redesign itself. Already, the involvement of human beings and human institutions in the production and design process is no longer always necessary.

To the extent that this is true – and it will be true to an even greater extent in the future – we will not be in a position to determine every aspect of the information environment. The technology will take over, acquiring a momentum of its own.

Self-reproduction and self-design

It is becoming common practice to write complex computer programs automatically, that is, using a program-writing program that accepts instructions expressed in a higher-level programming language and converts them into the forms required by the computer. The process is not so very different from that involved in using a team of human programmers to write a large suite of programs.

When a team of programmers is at work, the team leader and the system theorist who specifies the program-writing requirements will have very little idea of how the programs work; each individual programmer meets the specification he or she is given in his or her own way. Various precautions are taken to ensure that the different parts of the program will work together; for example, the program may be devided up into 'modules', so that the various parts of the program carry out specific operations and the links between them are minimized. There are also checks for correctness, to ensure that the individual programs do what they are supposed to do for all possible values of the data they handle.

In fact, under the combination of financial pressure, tight deadlines and human fallibility, the requirements for coherence between parts of the program are seldom fully satisfied. Correctness, in particular, cannot easily be determined except in simple cases, and most programs contain bugs as a result.

As far as both modularity and correctness are concerned, a program-writing program is likely to do a better job than a team of programmers. The system theorist's understanding of the program which results will be incomplete, but it is also incomplete when a human team is involved.

At the moment, program-writing programs and other methods for automating programming are being used to supplement, not to replace, the human programmer. Systems that will accept high-level specifications, and produce complex programs with minimal programming effort, are mostly advertised as aids to the programmer, releasing him or her from the chores of coding high-level instructions into lower-level languages. But potentially they could release the programmer from programming as it is generally understood.

In Chapter 9 we mentioned that there are now systems which use non-specialist statements from educators or authors to create programs that generate teaching strategies or hypotheses. They might, just as readily, generate designs or action

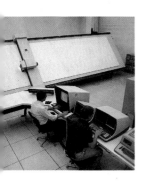

Computers are invading every aspect of design. This is the computerized drafting system used by Ford of Europe. Soon we will have computer programs that design computer programs. Will this create redundancies among the redundancy-creators?

strategies. The author, or team of authors, is interrogated, and has titular power of veto, and usually a more effective veto than that exercisable over the activities of a programming team. But although the author may have more power than a human team leader, he or she will have very little idea of what is, or is not, being vetoed, and very little idea as to how the program is satisfying the specifications given to it. With a program-writing program, therefore, total human involvement (as compared to a team leader's involvement) will be less.

More often than not, the author's responses to interrogation by the program do not afford control by veto; instead they give him or her the opportunity to alter specifications in subtle but important ways. Probably this is a good thing, as is the author's limited control overall. The consequences of altering specifications and objectives are seldom completely grasped. The idea that the author retains control of the program-writing program, or of its products, is illusory. The system controls itself.

There are also command and control systems in use today in which the behaviour of human commanders and the tactics they adopt form the statements of a higher-level language (no longer directly a programming language). These statements, in turn, are used to produce tactical programs that act as action generators if the people allegedly in charge of the system react too tardily to circumstances or go beyond the boundaries of safe operation.

As indicated in Chapter 5, there is no reason why statements in a high-level language need be statements by human beings. They need not be, and in fact are often not. Instead, they are statements generated by the operation of the system itself.

Exactly this kind of self-generating program is needed to design the networks constituting an information environment. The majority of existing networks could not have been devised without computer aid. Increasingly they are being devised by computer programs which incorporate humanly ambiguous requirements. The physical components of computers, microelectronic and biotechnological, are also being designed and made by computer programs. The manufacture of these components has to be automated; humans cannot achieve unaided the degree of precision and reliability required. And the assembly of components into computing or communication equipment can also be regulated without human intervention, using control systems and robots. The one time distinction between 'component' and 'assembly' is becoming arbitrary, if not pointless, in present-day technology.

To summarize, the idea that human beings determine exactly how processes in the information environment work, or exactly what the processes do, is questionable. To claim that we can determine what happens under all possible circumstances is spurious. Our statements merely influence operations and outcomes. Sometimes, they define them. They do not determine them.

Certainly, high-level statements are necessary in order to reproduce the information environment or to maintain it. However, they need not be human high-level statements. The job can be done better by the system itself. There is no reason, in principle, why the system should not act as a productive agent as well as a repairing one, generating design specifications to meet contingencies. Perhaps it had better do so if it is to survive, and (since we are rapidly coming to depend upon the system) if we are to survive. We ourselves are neither quick nor clever enough to do the job.

These notions are not novel. The concept of evolving and self-reproducing programs and machines dates back almost 30 years. Only recently, however, have these notions (and the realizations of them in the late 1950s and 1960s) become practical and economically viable in limited areas. The region of economic viability is nowadays increasing, as computing power becomes cheaper and as a wider range of options is recognized. Nevertheless, the full implications of this early work are still not widely acknowledged.

Controlled redundancy

There is an old and well tried design strategy which, up to a point, achieves the same objective as reproduction. In place of self-reproduction, the system is rendered highly redundant. Parts, functions, even the entire control and communication structure, are replicated in such a way that they can be substituted for one another if breakdown occurs.

A prime example of redundancy is a modern aircraft, a small and familiar part of the existing information environment. The aircraft is built with a very high degree of redundancy or replication; its control and communication systems are replete with microprocessors. Microprocessors all over the machine receive input from sensors which detect malfunctions, and control the substituting of malfunctioning components or operations with redundant capacity. The control and communication system of the aircraft is partly program-designed, and designed on the basis of fairly broad engineering models and specifications. The great safety of air travel is due to this design philosophy.

It would be false to say that the captain does not understand the aircraft, but it is true that he understands it only from an appropriate point of view, the one which permits him to control take-off and general course, deal with emergencies, receive signals from indicators of fuel level, engine temperature and so on, and act upon them. But he knows (at the time) very little about the state of the airframe or the minutiae of engine performance. He flies a machine buffered by control and communication systems.

Transition from an industrial environment to an informational environment constitutes a much wider and deeper revolution than earlier transitions. The revolution consists not of technological change or changes in employment patterns but of changes in the mental framework that makes our environment coherent to us. Our new mental framework encompasses different notions of the role of time, space, and dimensionality as a whole. It incorporates different ideas about the organization of knowledge, and about the meaning of learning and intelligence. Most of all, it allows for a different relationship between humans and machines.

We are already at the point where choosing to hand over control of part of our environment to computers is irrelevant. Whether or not our choice was conscious, that is what we have already done. We now live in an environment that we cannot hope to understand except from a specifically human perspective. This book provides part of that perspective. The other perspectives from which the environment can be both understood and controlled are not accessible to human beings. They are accessible to computers.

Unlike past environments the information environment is, and necessarily is, self-producing and self-reproducing, both by mechanisms that depend upon human beings, and by mechanisms that operate without the involvement of human beings.

The illusion of control. The information environment is so complex that even expert professionals cannot be said to control it in all its details.
Below left: a Tornado fighter plane, equipped with an advanced computer system that makes lightning decisions on the pilot's behalf. Below right: commercial aircraft have buffering and back-up systems to protect the pilot from information overload – he has enough to do coping with the instrument panel!

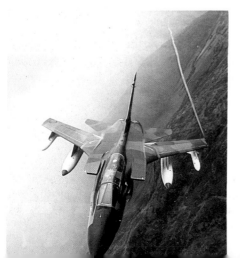

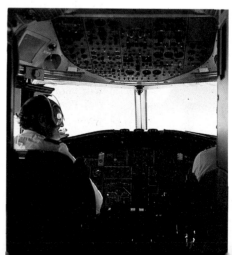

Chapter **11 THE BEST AND WORST OF POSSIBLE WORLDS**

The information environment described in the last chapter is the world today. Such a dramatic oversimplication is a valid picture only in the sense that a map of New York is a valid picture of New York. The map tells the truth, but the picture of New York that the map provides will probably not be the picture of New York that you have in mind. Your mental picture is probably much richer, full of images that have special meaning to you. It may also be less accurate. But your vagueness as to where Wall Street is, or how far the Statue of Liberty is from Manhatten Island, in no way invalidates your individual perspective.

To extend this analogy, the perspective from which we wrote the last chapter is in many ways similar to that of the mapmaker. The facts and figures we included prove that our perspective has some validity. But they provide a less than adequate picture of the modern world simply because their statistical accuracy does nothing to flesh out the description. If you are not accustomed to seeing the world as an information environment, we may have to work harder to change your perspective.

For that is our aim. We want to take your individual perspective on the modern world, and lay over it, like an extra filter, the concept of the information environment. The information environment does not skulk in a corner of the modern world. It is enmeshed with almost every aspect of it, and understanding its importance should change your entire concept of the world.

We are now going to offer a very individual picture of a world in which some of the potentialities opened up by information technology – psychological as well as practical – have been realized. It is a world which uses no technology that we do not already possess, or at any rate comprehend.

Is what follows our view of the world in AD 2000? Yes, in the sense that it extrapolates many trends and potentialities already outlined along paths we can reasonably expect to have travelled by the year 2000. No, in that we do not attempt to allow for the development of many other aspects of the modern world. Our world of AD 2000 is not a world in which the problems of nuclear war, over-population or racial problems are dominant. It is a world shaped by the information environment, in directions in which the current information tide seems to be carrying us.

AD 2000

Let us imagine the year AD 2000 has arrived. By now the information environment is part and parcel of general consciousness. Information, communication and control systems dominate common sense and reasonable ways of looking at the world. People are accustomed to them and make the fullest possible use of them.

Popular ideas of time and space have altered beyond recognition. So, too, has everyday existence. In AD 2000 duties which many people in 1980 regarded as irksome, such as going to the office or shopping, have changed their character entirely. As new dimensions have opened up to us, life has become much freer. There is an infinity of ways in which people can choose to run their lives and occupy themselves. Gordon Pask's life, as an academic offers one possible pattern; Susan Curran's life as a working mother another pattern.

The development of computing has led to a revolution in our concept of time. We no longer see time as we did, as a single track, heading in one direction only, straight for the future. Today Gordon and Susan conceive their lives as having a far more complex time structure, a structure which makes use of more than one dimension. We are now used, for instance, to living our lives in parallel, repeating parts of our own time pattern, and tying in to passages (not necessarily synchronous) from other people's lives.

The information environment has helped us to live out these new ideas. You can at any instant place yourself, by agreement, in contact with any number of immediate friends, and vice versa. You can retrieve the record of your own life, and in a sense relive it over any significant interval. With their consent, you can do the same with your friends' lives. This is seen as little different from accessing the many media channels currently available (up to 180 in London) or recording and retrieving their contents from video disc stores some time later.

Research has demonstrated the importance of bodily and personal rhythms, and the relative unimportance of a fixed diurnal scheme. Many people choose to adapt their patterns of work, play and sleep accordingly. Gordon has long opted to work mainly at night. Susan keeps more conventional hours to fit in with the demands of her family. Gordon and Susan communicate mainly by recorded messages; occasionally they compromise on a time for a videophone conversation or a face-to-face meeting.

Today we buy time as our parents used to buy accommodation, as space to live in. There are as many real time agents as real estate agents. The clock has certainly not lost all importance. Just as the clock in a computer plays a vital role as a scheduling agent, so the diurnal clock acts as a synchronizing factor in human life.

Space is seen from a wider perspective. Transportation is now seldom necessary to existence. Commuting, for instance, has become archaic. The development of a comprehensive distributed communications system has led to the dispersal of offices and their staffs; they are now splayed out across suburbia. Like Gordon and Susan, most employees of national or private enterprises work mostly in their own homes, for the communication links they require are fitted to any marketable house or rentable apartment. Fibre optic and waveguide channels are as common and as necessary as the telephone and television set of earlier years. Only the peripheral equipment – video displays, keyboards, facsimile devices for hard copying, local storage media, and other job-specific gadgets – is supplied by the employer.

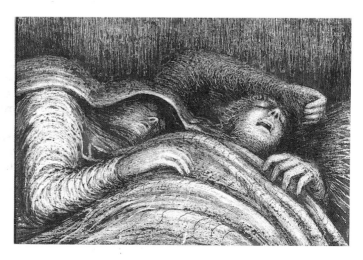

Travellers through time and space.

Gordon and Susan use the same communications system as the Prime Minister or the most junior clerk, but the devices they have attached to it are specific to them and their lines of work. In fact, configurations of personal equipment have become a meaningful, if rough-and-ready, index of job status. Gordon's system is unusually comprehensive but the equipment is functional rather than showy, as befits an academic. Susan does less computation, but rather more text editing; her word processing software is the best available.

People still meet their colleagues in the flesh from time to time. There are 'offices', social gatherings of reporters, programmers, politicians, control engineers, managers and word-processing executives adept at the complex arts of Xanadu. Here, too, status plays its part. Some offices vie for prestige with the principal London or New York clubs, and going to them serves much the same purpose as dropping in at one's club.

Shopping ceased to be a necessary feature of life some years ago. All household goods can be ordered and paid for via the communication system. Many recluses have all the necessities of life delivered to them and never venture beyond their front doors. Shops still exist because many people find visiting them a pleasurable leisure occupation. There has been a proliferation of specialist shops and restaurants, where people socialize as well as buy and eat. Gordon haunts the best bookshop in his neighbourhood; Susan still prefers to choose her own meat and vegetables, cheese and fruit.

In principle, Ted Nelson's Xanadu, which we discussed in Chapter 7, rendered the printed word redundant, and its 19-year-old successors have a haunting labyrinthine quality

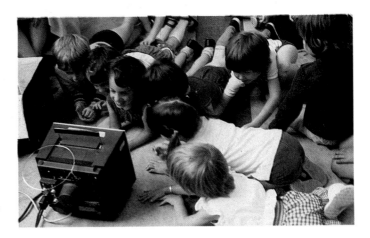

The process of education: a lifelong journey of discovery rather than a regime of fact between the ages of five and fifteen.

savoured by discriminating users. Not everybody enjoys navigating their way round the complex linkages, though; nor does ease of use of always win out over literary merit and sensuous delight. Contrary to some earlier forecasts, the printed word has never been more widely sought after, especially in well fashioned publications which count as works of art in their own right.

Education? Well, education is no longer synonymous with school and college. The information environment has become a major medium for inculcating facts and figures, and providing guidance and feedback. More sophisticated versions of the computer-aided learning systems described in Chapter 9 abound, and most people of all ages make use of them.

Youngsters today can learn their facts and figures at home, or in their friend's apartments, or (if they prefer it) around the globe. Adults learn too, continuously, and as a result our concepts of age and experience have undergone a metamorphosis. Youth is measured by the yardstick of a subject matter or a profession; Gordon is young in politics, though old in science. However, he is a specialist, and that is rare in this age. Most people have studied many skills and crafts, and all of us are able (even the specialists) to learn new ones. Susan is just beginning to learn Japanese, and in that she is still an infant.

Schools still exist. One of their major roles is one the computer cannot fulfil: to teach social skills, maturity and general demeanour. The computer's special role is to teach you how to learn. Learning to learn is the vital skill. Computers teach us to innovate, to take and combine different viewpoints, to find out information and fit it together. With this skill under their belts, youngsters are fitted for a lifetime of self-education.

The information environment has not decreased the theatre's popularity. The proscenium has always acted as an artificial boundary that accentuates the sense of close encounter, and it has survived the onslaught of television. Today, it competes successfully with holographic extravaganzas.

Transport is now a social rather than a solitary function. The microelectronic control systems found in cars of the 1980s have been greated refined and linked to a networked autopilot system. As a result, driving is peripheral activity, and for most of a journey driver and passengers can converse at leisure.

While private transport continues to flourish for business and pleasure, public transport systems have seen a great resurgence. Electric monorails are regular and seldom crowded; there is plenty of opportunity for travellers to exchange anecdotes, debate some common point of interest, or sit in comfortable solitude. In fact the monotrain is the meeting place most favoured by the intelligentsia bent upon serious discussions. Railway compartments, excepting those assigned to the shortest routes, are fitted with secretarial facilities, and much the same communication links as are found in the home can be rented on quite moderate terms. Journeying by air, by sea, or as the avant-garde prefer, beneath the sea, has much the same ambience as urban and inter-city travel.

Those who have a taste for travel and for socializing help to sustain the richest and in many ways the most respected citizens: those employed in the 'service' industries. Our lives would be impossible without the ticket lady at the station, the waiter on the train, the clerk at the bookshop, and the muscular crew who brought Gordon's equipment to his study when he was appointed to his post (and carried it with creditably little assistance from their robots). In recent years the service industries have become immensely sophisticated, and the continuing decline in the number of jobs available in manufacturing industry has meant that they can take their pick of staff. Because machines are the new servants, service has regained the dignity it used to have.

Work is no longer an essential activity. Our factories and farms are microprocessor-controlled and require only occasional human intervention and guidance. Of necessity we have evolved new methods of distributing goods and services. In Britain, negative income tax assures everyone of a basic income, while the rewards for working are less than they used to be. Other countries have adopted different systems. In the United States the free enterprise system is still predominant, while in the Eastern Block everyone is assured of at least a token job and an income to go with it.

Chess in the park, an aspect of the resurgence of all forms of al fresco socializing in the year 2000.

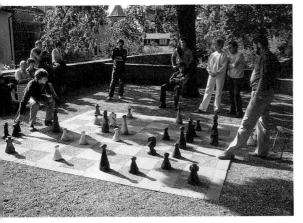
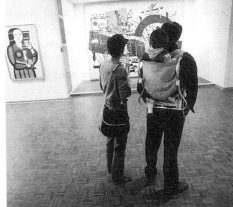

Though few countries force their citizens to work, many people still choose to work, and they show a commitment to their jobs comparatively rare a generation earlier. They are also highly and widely skilled. A transport system waiter is trained to perform the duties of a waiter, a chef or a manager, and is familiar with emergency procedures as well. The clerk in Gordon's favourite bookshop is a librarian, and has an encyclopaedic knowledge of science publications, but she also scolds him for his ignorance of Baudelaire in the original or Aristophanes in any form. The men who installed the electronic and other hardware in his study are not mere muscle men; they are well versed in electronics. They have to be, because their work depends on robot technology, and someone must maintain and not infrequently repair such mechanical servants.

Today almost all employment is seen as service. Male and female teachers, professors, scientists and artists are as much servants as male and female clerks, waiters, labourers and sanitary inspectors. So for that matter are the entertainers, the commentators and the gurus who appear as vivid holograms and talk through carefully positioned speakers in living rooms at large, providing a form of companionship (valued as such, whether the communication is one-way or two-way) to those who do not care to venture out of doors. The old distinction between white collar and blue collar has no meaning. Society is classless.

Changes in patterns of work in the home have led to wider changes in society. Few domestic chores are necessary today; domestic appliances have a high inbuilt level of intelligence. Microelectronic control systems run our homes. They even babysit, but our children still expect to see us, and not a robot, when they cry.

The cycle of work, play and domestic duty is no longer a binding limitation on most people's lives. As a result, the hard-and-fast male-female dichotomy is far less important than it was even in 1982, except of course for the most intimate biological particulars. Parents of young children, and those caring for the elderly and handicapped, are almost alone in being tied to a cycle of domestic activity. But even for them life is much less restricted than it was in the 1980s. Men as well as women have the time and the compassion to share the burden of caring for the helpless.

The word 'family' usually designates a wider group than parents and their immediate offspring. Although the institution has never been more revered, family memberships are seldom exclusive; people often belong to five or six families.

Marriage now means a contract of respect. It endures, like

Time, a commodity earned and saved by computer power; time to browse, to learn, to find yourself.

the family. But the observances of the 1980s – the daily split-role routine, the claustrophobic togetherness – are regarded as a strange psychopathology, with bitter symptoms that often kill that most precious gift, love.

The outer face, the surface, of the information environment is ribbed with furrows to accommodate the roles and institutions of this age. These roles and institutions have been shaped both by historical pattern and environmental accident, and by the oddities of human inclination. Activities once necessary for human existence have been transformed into optional pursuits. The niches provided by technology have been furnished by their inhabitants to provide a wide assortment of temporal and spatial satisfactions. Although there is no need to travel, and most of us know people who never move outside the confines of their apartments (for all it matters to their way of life, they might be living in Bel Air, Bangkok or Brussels), most of us like to venture into the outside world. Although the contents of almost any library could be projected over the translucent walls of our studies (any pair of books can be found displayed and compared within 30 seconds at most), we prefer to haunt bookstores and

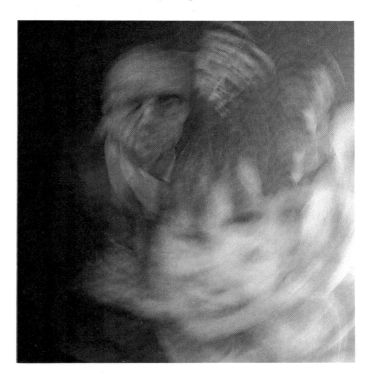

Everything spinning, complex, difficult to make sense of.

theatres and cafés. To a remarkable and perhaps unnerving extent, we are free, and need curtail that freedom very little in order to find congenial companionship.

These changes are well recorded. Often they are believed to be an inexorable consequence of melding humanity with a technological upsurge, but we suspect that happy circumstance, serendipity, played a part as well.

Influencing the future information environment

So far we have only looked at the outer face of the information environment. And from our very personal perspective, it is a smiling face, benevolent, almost Pickwickian. Penetrate below the surface, through the cracks to the interior, and we are not so sure about the smile. It is, after all, Gordon's job to work in the interior and Susan's to interpret its activity to the outside world. The 'inner face' could well turn ugly. We do not think it will, but we cannot be certain about it.

The unavoidable, maybe sinister, fact is this: the information environment builds itself and designs itself. No single person or group has a controlling option. The sheer complexity of the microcircuitry and communication nets of which this environment is made is well beyond the comprehension of even the most technically proficient of us. Automatic growth, design and repair are essential to the environment's survival, even to its existence. They were built into it of necessity; and the environment itself has now replicated and extended these facilities without deliberate human intervention.

Interior people like Gordon do a little tinkering and regulation, and people like Susan have a global overview of what goes on. But we are both well aware that increasingly we act as servants of (or, as our Union phrases it, 'consultants to') a self-repairing, self-evolving environment. To be truthful, we are not managers of the information environment; we have no illusions on that score.

Perhaps that is fortunate. A physicist does not and cannot know the state of every atom in a bagful of gas, let alone of every particle in a reactor. He is reasonably confident about some global rules, and how they will behave en masse. But if he tried to mess around at the atomic level, making sure that every single atom behaved predictably, he might well do more harm than good. So might we, if we relinquished our global overview and tried to interfere with the detailed happenings within microtechnology. Some of the happenings we have studied seem bizarre or misguided to us, but that may be because we cannot comprehend enough of the larger pattern to make sense of them. Try to change them, and we might find that they are vitally important. It seems safer to stick to our global perspective where, by and large, we can understand, predict, and partly influence what happens.

Earlier civilizations were concerned with mechanics and energy as limiting factors. They had to understand the laws of physics in order to progress, and so those laws seemed to be, and were, of primary significance. They stood out as salient to professionals and laymen alike. These laws remain substantially unchanged today. The law of energy conservation, for example, is still a solid, reliable rule of thumb. It does not matter to the mass of humankind going about its daily life that at the atomic level perpetual motion (prohibited by the law of energy conservation) is essential rather than impossible. But the educated person of today knows that we have lost the cosy conviction that such laws are immutable. Today we deal in probabilities, not in certainties.

The information environment has similar global principles, some of which we identify as laws. Like the laws of physics, they operate on a human scale and are virtually unaffected by our lack of certainty over goings-on at the micro level. It is these higher level principles that are of immediate concern today. We are still, to some limited extent, able to determine the information environment. We have a hand in choosing the roles it will obey as it evolves. So far, the environment is not quite given by nature, although very soon it will be for all practical purposes. At this point the members of our Union (the Union of Information Scientists) will, at best, be in the position of natural historians, specimen hunters who classify the anomalous species that inhabit the information kingdom.

Meanwhile, while we remain somewhere on the borderline between acting as 'consultants' to and 'servants' of the evolving information environment, there is an issue of professional conduct that has to be addressed, an ethical issue. The Union has adopted codes of good practice to help ensure that as global rules evolve into laws of nature, human values and preferences will remain enshrined in them. The important codes of practice can be expressed as conservation principles, not unlike the conservation principles of physics on which they were – not altogether consciously – based. They are four:

1. Conservation of concept sharing. This code states that, in any region, some concepts should be shared between human beings.

2. Conservation of concept creation. This means that innovation must always take place; our system of knowledge must always remain self-organizing.

3. Conservation of sufficient privacy to maintain individual identity, to ensure that individuals, like concepts, remain distinct from each other.

4. Conservation of balance. The rate at which ideas and concepts become rigid and ossified shall not exceed the rate at which new concepts are evolved.

Perhaps more significantly, the Union takes it for granted that the information environment will not only evolve but also grow. We accept that it will become increasingly pervasive and that the power of its microelectronic controllers, and its capacity for data storage, will increase. At the same time the rate of communication, meaningful or not, will increase. This is not dogma, but fact. It has happened and will happen.

As we look further into the future, it is more and more apparent that what will mould our development as human beings is not technological determinism but human choice. The information environment is already able to support a wide variety of different lifestyles. As its power grows – and we take it for granted that it must – the range of lifestyles it can accommodate will grow too.

Let us now look further into the future, and alert you to some implications of the information environment beyond AD 2000. Our main concern is to outline not technical developments but psychological ones. And as a vehicle for evaluating these future scenarios, we shall use the Union Code outlined above, with its criteria of concept sharing, concept creation, privacy and balance.

We believe an information environment could satisfy all of these criteria if it consisted of a population of machines, some interfaced with human beings. By population of machines, we mean what we meant in Chapter 4: a linked group of independent self-organizing machines capable of conflict as well as conflict resolution.

Some of the distinctions made in Chapters 5 and 6 are also worth reiterating at this point, because they affect our use of language. For example, communication (a facility with the same neutral connotation as computation, control or data storage) is not the same as conversation, in which concepts are shared and created. And again, data storage is not the same commodity as knowledge. An information environment, in which it is taken for granted that communication will increase, could just as easily impede as promote concept sharing and creation.

The distinction between knowledge and information also bears reiteration. Take a mass of computer printout, or an afternoon of accelerated viewdata reception; both provide information from data storage, but that information is as likely to overwhelm as to inform the recipient. Even if it does inform, neither the stacked-up printout nor the flux of images is knowledge. They may aid the acquisition of knowledge or hinder it, but the mere presence of items of data is not knowledge.

Examples of how concepts are not shared, and how knowledge is not acquired, are commonplace and obvious. But there are other characteristics of an information environment that have more subtle, less understood, and equally paradoxical effects. These we hope to convey through the five scenarios which follow.

Scenes from a future time

Each of the scenarios given below is shaped by obedience or disobedience to the codes stated on page 198. In each case, we shall point out which codes are kept and which broken. We intend these as forecasts, as informed prophecies if you like. If our lens seems deliberately distorting, we can only retort that to us they are all valid perspectives on reality. They are no more deliberately science-fictional than any other forecast. They are the possible consequences of satisfying or not satisfying the codes we have outlined, and of the overall rapid increase in the power of technology. In fact, our forecasts are very conservative, for they rely only upon principles of cognition and computation well established at the time this book was written.

Too much togetherness

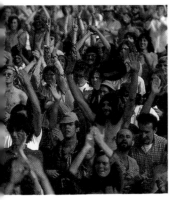

Chiefly flourishing in Southern California the cult-like, often orgiastic Togetherness Movement becomes established in Europe in about 2005. Here, it takes on a distinctive Old World flavour, tinged with the fundamentalism and back-to-nature fervour that go hand in hand with taking things quite literally. Apart from these propensities, the movement employs encounter techniques in order to achieve its aim that everyone share their psyche with everyone else. The Togetherness Party mobilizes and wins power with the slogan 'Equal Opportunity to Communicate'.

An ordinance of 18 May 2020 asserts that all people shall be equidistant. A typical statute (66574) prohibits impediments to communication by physical boundaries of any kind. Property developers leap upon the bandwagon, and construct estates full of transparent and unsoundproofed buildings. Towards July 2020 the occupants of these legal but diaphanous structures express opposition to the whole idea, transparent boudoirs in particular causing them great embarrassment. Later in the month several apartment blocks collapse — few injuries are sustained since at that stage there are few remaining occupants. James

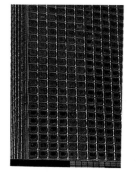

An apartment block built in accordance with Statute 66574.

Sharing	Yes
Creation	No
Privacy	No
Balance	No

One of the rash of Anti-Togetherite demonstrations that marked the year 2020 (official photograph)

Merrivale, President of the European Architects' Union, pronounces the style 'ugly, unsafe and frankly ludicrous', and the Chairman of the British Architectural Association concurs, adding: 'The provisions of Statute 66574 cannot be satisfied in the three-dimensional space used by architects'. On 17 July zealot Togetherites bulldoze the greater part of that physical southern English boundary, Milton Keynes, and on 18 July a comparably violent incident eliminates Hamburg in West Germany.

These civil disturbances provide an excuse for the government to change policy. 'Of course one cannot be equidistant in three dimensions', pronounces the Minister for the Environment, 'but the information environment has endless dimensions'. After some consultation about what this gnomic utterance means, the government revises Statute 66574 to read: 'Any opaque obstacle, wall, floor or ceiling must be penetrated by at least 120 MHz fibre optic cabling' and make provision for 'touch sensors, full holographic equipment, projective test facilities, and other means to facilitate soul searching'.

Attitude research is carried out which reveals that people do not, in fact, soul search even under these propitious conditions. There follow until 2026 no less than five 'togetherness promot-

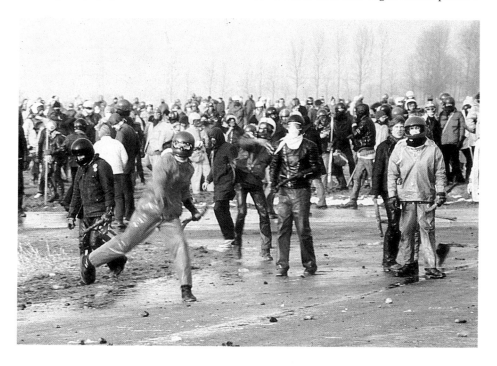

Sharing	Yes
Creation	Yes
Privacy	No
Balance	No

ing' Acts. One provides that any closed space in which no sharing of inner secrets can be detected be immediately filled with a noxious odour; another that any occupant of such a space be given painful, but harmless, electrical stimulation.

Despite these government initiatives, by 2026 no conversation takes place whatsoever. Since everyone is alike there are no concepts, personal or otherwise, left to share; there is no need to talk. People have adapted to the continual punitive stimulation, and have come to regard it as the one contenting feature of life.

Sharing	No
Creation	No
Privacy	No
Balance	No

Or nearly so. Thanks to some maverick legislators who are not yet completely silent, it becomes possible to buy privacy in much the same way as one used to buy silence from a juke box – by selecting a silent record. As a result, the population divides into 'hermits', who are said to think and even dream (there is ample evidence that they occasionally share concepts, too), and 'replicas', who exchange signals which are meaningless except as an indication of sameness.

Micro-freak societies

I t is AD 2002. First children, and then adults, have become addicted to microprocessors of the kind available in 1982, but with greater storage capacity and better peripherals. Their addiction to peeky, linearized images of reality is so strong that when they do converse (and micro freaks are notoriously taciturn) they do so through their micros in programmatic terms. Although the information environment is capable of handling much richer images, the micro freaks prefer to transmit arid program listings accompanied by a few explanatory notes. It is true that people meet for hasty meals, and to purchase computer books or mind-boggling volumes of recreational mathematics. But even face-to-face transactions are jargon-laden at best, and usually monosyllabic.

Sharing	Yes
Creation	Yes
Privacy	Yes
Balance	No

By 2020, the habits of 2002 have become even more deeply ingrained. Mostly people engage in games, problem solving and abstract invention. They appear to interact through their games, although no meaningful interpretation of these interactions can be found, except in terms of empty symbols and formal systems of numbers.

People do not go out. They eat in their dens. In contrast, the information environment is busy executing programs and forming patterns of immense complexity and – if they could be perceived – profound beauty. Perhaps people see beauty in their abstract world, through the tiny window of their computers. It is difficult to gauge their attitudes, for only a few will reply to questions.

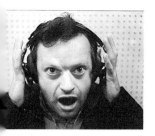

Garth G., chairman of
the Young Micro-Freaks,
born 1999.

Q *Why don't you go out?*
R *Why should I?*
Q *There's a café round the corner.*
R *Eh? Round the what? Yes, I see what you mean,
orthogonally, in a plane of Euclidean three space...*
Q (slightly embarrassed) *Ordinary space.*
R *Not ordinary, quite unusual. There aren't enough
dimensions, nothing like 100. Anyhow, I'm usually in
Reimann space. (At this juncture, the questioner prepares to
leave, and asks the time. The respondent is puzzled.)*
R *There isn't any time... just instructions TRUP or TRPR.
Oh, but you mean order... yes... between 2005 and 2060, but
that's pretty stupid.*

The world is a timeless mathematical labyrinth. Its aesthetic
is the music of the spheres, held captive by the timeless
symmetries of pure cognition stripped of feeling. It is a crystal-
line world. The only motion is governed by an order of program
execution.

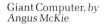

Giant Computer, by
Angus McKie

Q *What is life?*
R *Thought.*

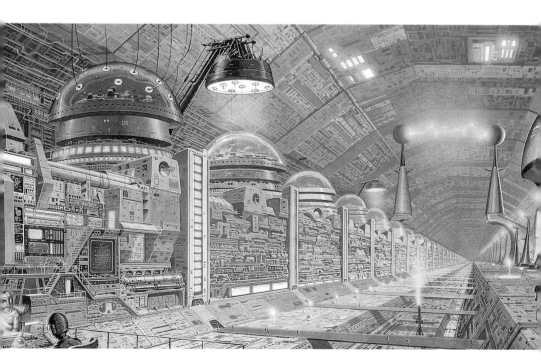

Anthill cultures

These interesting cultures, so named because of their superficial resemblance to an anthill or termite mound, differ in one fundamental way from the micro freak civilization. Anthill citizens are sadly uniform; they abhor deviance, and they have no pretensions to abstraction. The abstract micro freaks, on the other hand, concealed whatever deviation form the norm they possessed (they are all eccentrics) as an arid kind of creativity.

Early in their development anthill people differentiate into a 'motile' group and a less numerous 'cell dweller' group. The motiles, mostly members of our own Union, scutter around the information environment in a ritual frenzy of reconstruction and repair. The cell dwellers, probably because they have been genetically engineered to do so, remain contentedly static in their cells. All their needs and desires are satisfied automatically, with the indirect but conscious connivance of the motiles. Each cell dweller is devoted to a 'job' that closely resembles the jobs handled by the earliest computer centres. Cell dwellers are quite loquacious when it comes to job-oriented dialogue. They say their life consists of 'decision making' via the information interfaces with which their cells are equipped. Because job-specific messages transmitted between cells are easy to intercept, each cell dweller believes he or she is a decision maker of some importance.

Q *Do you take responsibility for all of these decisions?*
R *Oh no, the caucus takes responsibility.* (The caucus is an anthill idiom for a committee.)

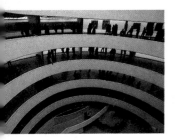

Above: one of many continuous spiral structures designed for 'motiles'.

Right: a hilltop Anthill community.

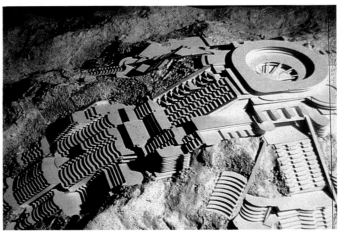

An impartial observer soon becomes aware that a cell dweller's belief in his or her importance in the world is spurious. Cell dwellers handle bits of business and do routine checks, the kind of operations which in the mid-1970s used to be called 'noise'. There is continual chatter but no decisions are ever made either by individual cell dwellers or by caucuses of them. This aspect of their culture is supported by further enquiry.

Q *Where is knowledge?*
R *In our environment.*

Sharing	Yes
Creation	No
Privacy	Yes
Balance	No

Which can be construed as meaning that cell dwellers lay no claim to having knowledge themselves. Nor, for all their chatter, do they constitute a real society.

An outsider with a yen for symmetry might ask about the motiles' view of the world. Answers are hard to get. Motiles long ago adapted to pure movement, and it is absurd to think of asking one of them anything.

A note on archaeology

Archaeologist Giulia Marina, in a commentary written in 2970, writes with acumen about these varied species of micro men and women. She is especially concerned about the periodic fall and reincarnation of each civilization.

Much of Marina's text would be familiar to an archaeologist of 1980 or earlier. She is on the look-out, as they were, for any hump-shaped mound on a Greek Island or in the Middle East, that may yield, on excavation, cities built on cities, the artefacts of cultures long past. Yet, unlike her older colleagues, Marina is not offended by detritus placed upon the mound by people in the neighbourhood. She takes it as a sign of continuity in life. And if she walks through Acre, say, on alleys whittled out of the Acre of years ago, she literally relives the lives of the Phoenicians, the Crusaders, the Turks. Their cultures are revitalized by her ramble through them.

Some of Marina's hypotheses about the wax and wane of micro man would be familiar to 1980 archaeologists. They are of the kind that were employed to explain the sudden fall of the first palace cultures of Knossos and Phaestos on Crete (this was attributed in 1980 to a tidal wave, the aftermath of a volcanic outburst which formed the islands of Santorini).

Marina notes 'a certain contradiction in the phasic developments of micro men of different species'. She comments that 'biotechnology provided a computing medium of greater power than microelectronics, although in many excavations we find them mingled. In terms of cost effectiveness the least expensive component for the information environment was the human

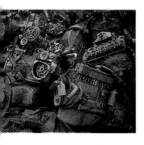

Excavations on a site near Frankfurt, Northern Empire. The primitive engineering methods suggest a wastage date somewhere between 1980 and 1990.

being: virtually costless, especially if engineered to eat less food and occupy less space. Many civilizations of micro men must have recognized the fact, and there is ample evidence that some acted upon it. In this lies one possible explation for the curious periodicities we all observe'.

Our species

The main distinctions between the world of 2120 and the world of 2000 are not to be found in changed technology or changed behaviour. The distinctions are between prevalent attitudes and beliefs, between the different ways in which we look at ourselves and our environment. Some people in 2000 half perceived the innovations that made Togetherness, Freakdom, and Anthill dwelling possible, but at that stage they had a narrow view of the potentialities. Now, our vision of things is far wider.

It is hard to pinpoint in exactly what ways our vision is wider, because where thinking people of 2000 would have justified their arguments by proceeding from cause to effect, currently we do not seek to justify things by sequential reasoning. We juxtapose and compare perspectives, each of them having various dimensions; some of these perspectives have many kinds of dimensionality, some none at all. This mode of thinking is different from that of our predecessors, but is neither better nor worse. On reflection it is perhaps better because it helps us to avoid the cultural excesses that overwhelmed the Freaks and Anthill dwellers.

We have, for example, overcome the almost obsessive and damaging tendency to give names only to heads and bodies (one reason, we suspect, for our species' early pre-occupation with dancing figurines and humanoid robots). Riding on the technology of 2120 (not so different from the technologies latent in 2000), the average person is usually distributed across the information environment. Anne, Jo or Bill may literally inhabit many places at once; many people may also be in the same place - for instance in one brain - at once. But what is more important is the absence of an imperative. No individual is *obliged* to be splayed across his or her friends. No one is *forced* to concentrate their being in one head, either their own or any other.

It has always been natural for media interviewers to focus on sex whenever they are in difficulties. Let us listen to a human being of 2120 from the perspective of an interviewer of our own time, a time in which sex seemed such a skin-to-skin and down-to-earth affair.

Sharing	Yes
Creation	Yes
Privacy	Yes
Balance	Yes

Q You said you can make love to John, even love him, even live with him, without either of you moving?

Anna Yes, surely.

Q In a poetic... er... Platonic sense?

Anna Not particularly.

Q I mean, can you copulate, have sex... that kind of thing?

Anna Oh yes, that is quite usual.

Q And with Alan, or (coyly consulting a notebook) Peter?

Anna Of course. I love them immensely. They are all very much a part of me, and I am very much a part of them. The arrangement is convenient – they can be all over Europe, or I can, it doesn't matter.

Q (coming down to brass tacks). Exactly how do you make love in different places without moving?

Anna You ought to know that. Plants make love at a distance, without moving... they have many ways of doing it. We have many more, indefinitely many – it's up to us to choose.

Q But how do you choose the most efficient way?

Anna What a stupid question. Efficiency kills love... don't be silly.

Q But isn't this environment boring, staying at home and sharing concepts and reproducing?

Anna You asked a practical question, can I make love without moving, and I said 'yes'. Do you really think that 'can' means 'must' and that it's the only thing to do? Jaime took me out to dinner last week, in Acapulco, and I stayed on at his place. We both like travelling and had a wonderful couple of days in Mexico. You do have a blinkered view of things...

As it happens, the interview of which this is a transcript was deemed unsuitable for a family audience and was not transmitted until some years later. Had it been transmitted, and buttressed by the technology existing even then, much human misery might have been avoided at very small cost. In the old days people took themselves too earnestly. Good heavens, they used to die for love!

Is this the future - any of it? Or perhaps at different times in our species' ongoing history, all of it? We can make no pretence to know. We do know, though, that to us these are some of the scenarios possible in a world ruled by the micro as well as by the human species.

Chapter **12** METAMORPHOSIS OF MACHINES & MAN

The proposition that microcomputers are only small-scale computers is not entirely true. For with the power that microelectronics, biotechnology and other exotic technologies bring, comes the possibility that the simple computational devices we examined in Chapter 1 may metamorphose into something else.

Emerging into a new world

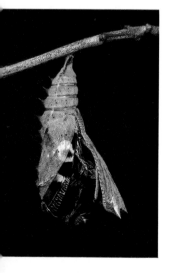

Let us imagine a system, of a type as yet unstated, but bootstrapped by the technology that is channelled at the moment into micros. Suppose that such a system could be like a brain, and carry out operations that are mindful. Impossible? Current research into artificial intelligence, and the concept of a population of computers liberated from the serial straightjacket of conventional computing, carry this notion well into the realm of the probable.

A probability of this kind inevitably induces a kind of pre-metamorphic shock. The most frightening and shock-provoking aspect of metamorphosis is not the fear of mental castration that we looked at in Chapter 2, but fear of the great unknown. It is the fear that would face tadpoles, if they had the wit, presented with the prospect of froghood; or a caterpillar, told a tale of butterflies.

How do we view ourselves and our society, confronted with the prospect of being transformed beyond our imaginations? Have we wit enough to fear the future? Have we wit enough to overcome that fear?

It would make good sense for us to be afraid if we were convinced that the proper habitation for mind must always be the human brain. On the contrary, there is good reason to believe that habitations of the sort in which the mind can live, grow and undergo transformation without loss of personality, will soon exist in some profusion. They are the habitations offered by the information environment, described in its infancy in Chapter 10 and envisaged in its full flowering in Chapter 11. And with these habitats, these technology niches, will come a metamorphosis for the human species that parallels the metamorphosis of machines. The interplay between the two species will create an information environment that is a fit and mutual habitation for both human and non-human minds.

Is there a sinister price to be paid for this post-metamorphic Utopia? The price might be alienation, alienation between persons, or alienation between persons and the information environment. Another sinister possibility might be a world in which machines are beyond our control, working not in our best interests but against them. We do not deny these possibilities, but we believe they can be avoided.

Reductionist man and his antithesis

In our introduction we commented on a development in thought and natural philosophy even more important than the emergence of computation. This was the human propensity to view reality as a linear, sequential progression of events. This view coloured the development of mathematics and dominated the mathematical concept of time.

In one way or another, depending upon their different persuasions, mathematicians as well as natural philosophers, and the scientists who came later in history, imaged time as though it were the counting of instants (knots) along a line (a piece of string). This image, prettied-up and formalized, came to permeate the design of standard computing machines.

The image is correct enough. It is seductive in its appeal to neatness and simplicity. We do not deny its correctness, nor do we deny that it often seems, and sometimes is, valid to say that we attend to one thing at once, one thing after another. However, we do deny the universality of this idea. For it pertains to the limited sphere of deductive, and some kinds of inductive, inference to which computer scientists have for the most part restricted themselves. It does not apply to reasoning by analogy, or to reaching novel hypotheses, or to creativity, or to invention.

We can, if we want to, hold the view that consciousness, existence, flows like a river. But we can only do so if we accept that the vortices and eddies, the events of which it is constituted, possess a varied dimensionality. A single dimension is simply not rich enough as a description of a river.

We can implement a version of a multi-dimensional world view as a model in a computer, using complex manipulations which some would claim to encompass both thought and consciousness. It would entail what Douglas Hofstadter (in *Gödel, Escher, Bach:An Eternal Golden Braid*) calls a 'vortex' of computer programs, each acting simultaneously upon others lower in a hierarchy during their execution.

It is generally assumed in such a model that the operation of each programmed loop, and the interaction of the many loops, takes place as though co-ordinated by a synchronizing signal. This view approaches reductionism, the belief that the action of any system can be expressed as the sum of the action of its parts.

Yet it is possible to produce a quite different model of thought and consciousness. This other model takes a holistic view of things. It assumes that several foci of attention coexist, each with its own autonomous and potentially independent clock and counter. Each focus embodies at least one loop-like organization, and each is a possible world of action, or a person, or an institution. The co-ordination of the clocks and counters, if it occurs, occurs by virtue of the whole process rather than according to predetermined rules. A system modelled in this way is truly self-organizing. It is this co-ordination of potentially independent units which is consciousness, a property of the whole and not of the parts. The degree of consciousness is determined by the degree of co-ordination. The contents of consciousness are the loop-like organizations shared between the different foci.

A world of many dimensions impossible to properly describe or understand piecemeal.

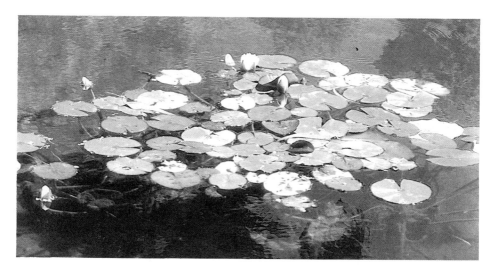

If the synchronizing operations which are generally built into the first model are removed, then in effect the first model acquires the characteristics of the second. Instead of parallel processing, however complex, we end up (in Hofstadter's phrase) with 'strange loops and tangled hierarchies' that really exist. But the interaction between them, which constitutes the consciousness of the system, is no longer describable in reductionist terms.

These views are not mutually exclusive. One or the other, or both, could reasonably be maintained, and we have used both models in this book. But if both of them were denied, then events would not be conscious events; strictly and surely they could not be. The fallacy of supposing that there might and could be conscious events without an interaction system of some kind is responsible not only for shaping the form of computers in a way which excludes consciousness from consideration, but also for the ignoring of consciousness and allied phenomena by most scientific psychologies.

The linearity or seriality of temporal events that underpins the reductionist orientation of the first model is useful if one is mainly concerned with deductive mental operations, and if these operations are considered to be the predominant mental processes. The idea of seriality is misleading if, at the other extreme, one believes that learning and doing are essentially creative. Creativity and invention entail not only self-reference, production and reproduction, but also the juxtaposition of conflicting perspectives and the resolution of conflicting situations. The latter activities are not compatible with the idea of seriality. They are better captured by the holistic model.

Throughout this book our stance has been that mental activities are primarily inventive or creative – learning entails discovery, and action involves imagination, analogizing and venturing into the unknown. In principle we believe that individuals could converse creatively through the medium of a population of computers, a system connected in a way that allows for both conflict and conflict resolution. This is the sort of system that microelectronics has made possible.

Our conjecture is that humanity is at a point of departure, on the verge of a revolution in thought, where the linear-destructive paradigm is being replaced by a paradigm of creativity as the main pursuit of humankind.

Models of mind

Let us make a detour and consider how human intelligence and machine intelligence fit in with some of the ideas put forward by two apparently opposite schools of thought in experimental psychology: the behaviourists, and the cognitive scientists. Oddly enough, both exclude consciousness from the field of scientific enquiry; their logical framework prohibits either explanation or demonstration of the nature of consciousness, thought and allied phenomena.

Behaviourism holds that an organism (generally thought of as a person, though nearly all behavioural data have been obtained from animal experiments) is well demarcated from its environment. Stimuli, externally as well as internally generated, provoke responses which form sequences of behaviour. According to behaviourist principles, all that can or need be known in scientific psychology can be gathered from an analysis of sequences of behaviour under controlled conditions. To put it very simplistically, the organism is seen as a 'black box', as having input and output and a defined boundary.

The trouble is that people do not normally live in experimental situations which can be controlled or manipulated. Moreover people only take part in experimental situations because they agree to do so. But black boxes cannot agree! Behaviourist studies cannot, therefore, say anything about agreement, mind, consciousness or other subjective matters.

In contrast, cognitive psychology is concerned with mental and symbolic events. It starts out with a model, which may be constructed to image experience, or constructed according to reports, protocols or introspection. Now, by far the most versatile and elegant medium for modelling a complex process is a computer program. For the cognitive psychologist the use of such a program is both liberating and dangerous. Up to a point, the psychologist is at liberty to interpret a model, albeit in the form of a computer program, as representing mental conditions. Executing the program under different conditions may allow the psychologist to predict possible behaviours with accuracy. None of this commits the psychologist to the mistaken view that the states of a computer are states of mind, or that program execution is more than a simulation. Nevertheless the distinction may be forgotten; a program that represents a model of states of mind may be taken to be an actual model. If that happens, the cognitive scientist, for all his or her sophistication and apparent mentalism, becomes shackled by the constraints built into computers, constraints that are directly analogous to the self-imposed restrictions of the behaviourist.

Obviously both behaviourists and cognitive scientists do observe and say a great deal about consciousness, and they are well aware that the functional boundaries of a subject rarely coincide with the biological carapace. One person's brain cannot be viewed in isolation from its extension into other people's thoughts, or even into computers. But these observations do not belong to the official and objective picture common to strict behaviourism and pure cognitive science.

The position we adopt in this book is described by de Gelder and others as 'interactionist', because the phenomena of interest to us are intended actions or transactions consciously performed. In fact Gordon Pask is responsible for a brand of interactionism called Conversation Theory, which has been formalized and tailored to deal with transactions involving computers and information systems. The bias is admitted, but we believe the theory does not go against a commonsense view of sentient beings. It enables us to regard people and the perspectives they entertain not only as discrete units, but also as existing in a matrix of other perspectives or social institutions – corporate, political, religious, stylistic, educational and philosophical.

Micro men in psychology

A few years ago behaviourism and pure cognitive science (not cognitive psychology) dominated the intellectual scene in Britain and the United States (other European and American countries have more liberal traditions). At that time, the position we have adopted would have seemed utterly alien to the mainstream. Now the situation is different. Other schools of psychology and sociology are serious contenders with behaviourism for the status quo, and a pure cognitive science is giving way to a genuine cognitive psychology. An interactionist position is no longer heretical.

There is, for example, growing appreciation of American psychologist George Kelly's theory of 'personal constructs', that corresponds closely to the 'memorable concepts' we described in Chapter 3. In Kelly's theory, people are characterized by an organization of core constructs closely akin to the participants in a dialogue. People act like personal experimenters or explorers, construing the world in a personal way but entering into agreement over some of its features.

Another compatible theory is the 'interpersonal psychology' of British psychiatrist R. D. Laing, which is particularly concerned with acts of agreement – with agreeing to disagree, and how one person understands why and how there is agreement or disagreement with another person. Like the clinically oriented psychologies of Freud and Jung, both Kelly's and Laing's theories deal, necessarily, with consciousness and awareness of 'self' and 'other'. Acts of agreement, construing, understanding and so on can be quantified and therefore belong to the domain of scientific psychology. Through a new generation of psychology theorists, incuding many others besides Kelly and Laing, we are beginning to see the reshaping of our perception of the world in the image of micro man. The crude image of people as machines, people as creatures explicable within a simple, bounded, serial framework, is being overtaken by the image of both people and machines as far more rich and strange.

A holistic view
of the information
environment

The same reductionist attitude that has limited our view of consciousness and thought has hindered people from a full appreciation of the developing information environment. The information environment is not so much hidden as not perceived. The single-minded reductionism of nineteenth century science and technology served us well in the industrial stage of evolution, but it has conditioned us to think in terms of bits and pieces.

We must discard this atomistic, dissecting-room stance not because it has no validity, but because it has no relevance. Imagine a bargain between the joint owners of a motor car. They are to share the automobile half-and-half. They debate whether to bisect the vehicle nose to tail, or left to right across its midriff. Lamentably, neither remnant can be driven. The feature of the car which makes it a mode of transport cannot be exploited by taking the car to bits; it resides in a combination of the bits.

So it is with the information environment. It resembles the polyps in a coral reef, each building its limestone dwelling but each interacting with hundreds of neighbours through filaments which ramify throughout the reef, co-ordinating its activity. The only difference is that the information environment is widely spread. Communication and control are distributed. Not only does this mean that there have to be lots of different micro-processors connected by links and channels, but also that it is pointless to ask which bit senses, which bit computes, which bit takes action, and which bit delivers messages.

Interlude:
the boundaries
of scepticism

Long ago the late Professor A.M. Low employed Gordon Pask briefly each year to expurgate those entries from the annual exhibition of the British Society of Inventors and Patentees that were ingeniously concealed perpetual motion engines, and thus unpatentable, since perpetual motion contravenes well-established laws of nature.

Most of the illegitimate entries could easily be excluded as brash or uninformed, occasionally tragic, often comical, essays in getting something for nothing. But some, at least as ideas or designs on the drawing board, were not so naive. The question 'Is that a perpetual motion machine?' became 'Is that a machine?' If not – if it did not work within the popular scientific frame of reference – then it could not constitute an entry. This or that design, even though manifestly unpatentable as a mechanical, chemical or electrical gadget, might have worked inside a different frome of reference, inside some other consensually agreed structure with laws different from those of elementary machines, electricity, or chemistry, and tested by different consensually agreed methods of observation.

A hesitancy of just this kind is called for when thinking of systems that are neither orderly computers nor biological sludges, but environments made of computer-technology fabric in which minds might metamorphose and grow.

At the end of the day the patent laws, the laws of nature, and the tests of factuality which establish these laws, are all inventions of the human mind. Metamorphosis of that mind could give rise to quite different frames of reference.

The control of unavoidable trends

Increasingly, the trend of the information environment is towards literal self-reproduction rather than the similar but longer used philosophy of redundancy of parts and functions. We believe this trend is unavoidable as the information environment becomes more pervasive and resilient. In fact we welcome this trend. It leads towards information structures that are less cumbersome and more versatile than structures based on redundancy alone, but such structures do not readily yield to analysis by reductionist methods. This is why the information environment is hard to come to grips with and hard to govern. Does this matter?

The human race does not have a particularly good record when it comes to managing environments that are neither fully appreciated nor fully open to reductionist analysis. For example, the management of the ecology was incompetent until people were forced to recognize that a global rather than an analytical approach was mandatory. That point was hard to reach. But from there we moved on to cleaning rivers, reducing city smog and rendering the Great Lakes habitable again. People became ecology conscious.

More than once in recent years the power supply for the East Coast of the United States has broken down, catastrophically. The designers claimed to understand the workings of the system they created, but though they may have understood the parts they manifestly failed to understand the whole.

In the light of such obvious failures, it may be wise for us to hand over certain productive capabilities, as well as self-reproductive capabilities, to an evolving information environment. Not that we have much option in the matter, for these

The natural world,
precious and
irreplaceable, and
coming under
increased pressure.

Inset: control room in a
modern power station.
Where are the human
controllers?

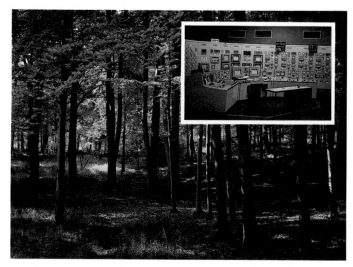

processes are already intimately bound up with each other. We are already living in an information environment which is both productive, reproductive, and unavoidably evolving.

Opting out

I s it too late to put the clock back? We believe it is. An attempt to dispense with the aid of machines on a large scale, or to restrict further development, is unlikely to lead to an arcadian idyll, Moreover, we believe that such an attempt is unnecessary. The flexible information environment avoids most of the shortcomings associated with earlier stages of computerization – the inexorable rule of the clock, the drive towards centralization. There is no prescription against decentralization and local autonomy in the age of micro man. Pockets of a de-informationalized society may survive, just as some remote areas have succeeded in sustaining an agricultural society throughout the age of industrialization.

We live in an
information
environment, but the
pre-information society
still survives.
Below: modern data
terminal, Australian
style. Below right:
visual display units,
Pakistani style.

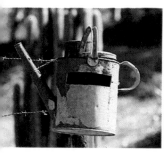

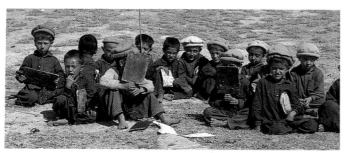

But most communities – particularly large prosperous ones – have no choice in the matter. They must opt in. The sooner this fact and its consequences become part of our consensual reality, the better for everyone.

Opting in

Are we poised to take another 'giant step' forward?

And so we come back to the scenarios of Chapter 11, to the alternative results of different strategies of opting in. Our first account, of AD 2000, was contrived to give a fresh view of things just as they are. It is a collation of personal and

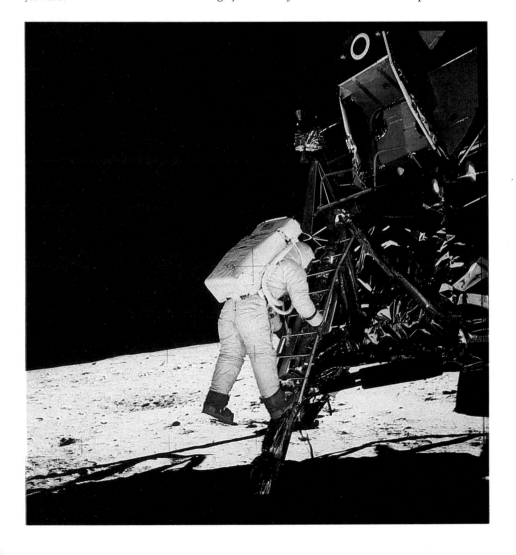

often vivid impressions garnered from all over the industrial world. We tried to look at existing realities and relevant styles of life. We tried to be sober, not bizarre. Only minor extrapolations entered into the composition, so we placed it 20 years hence.

Our forecasts are forecasts only. As you might suppose, we have personal faith in the last one, which we called 'our species'. We believe it is a desirable future and one we can genuinely hope to achieve. The image is not too far from the kind of image entertained by any thoughtful person, and many a poet, today or a century ago or longer in the past, or in the future.

We need to acquire a breadth (or is it laterality?) of vision, the kind of vision that the ancients called wisdom. We need a kind of amity, combined with the will to explore and the knowledge that no adventure ends or ever can do. And for that we need a broad perspective.

Stormy skies above, and we are earthbound yet. But we can reach out . . .

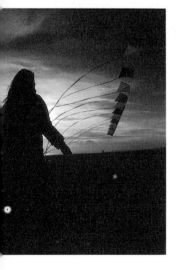

Such a perspective is what we hope this fancified, computer-ridden, but living world will give us all. It will teach us not to limit apprehension to a narrow aperture. We can live in many worlds at once, for 'once' has lost its customary meaning.

This freedom will mean that the mandate 'Choose a corner' or 'Choose a lifestyle' is no longer compulsive or compulsory. Few choices will be irrevocable. The information environment will support a multitude of different patterns of living and permit us to change our lifestyle if we find we do not like it.

Does this mean that we should opt out of controlling the growth of the information environment? No, but it does mean that we need only attempt to control it at certain levels and from certain perspectives. At other levels the information environment can do the job better itself. Our choices will not need to be detailed technical ones, a switch on or off here, a communication line open or closed there. Rather they will be choices at the macro level enshrined in the Union Code of the year AD 2000: sharing of concepts, creation of new ideas, maintenance of individual identity, and continuation of a sense of balance and order. It is to such laws that we must look if we are to influence the evolution of micro man, or, for that matter, to survive at all.

INDEX

Credits/Photographs

Advisory Unit for Computer-based Education Peter Andrews 163 *All Sport* Tony Duffy 64 *Apex Photos Ltd.* 92 top *Apple Computers (U.K.) Ltd.* 25 *Ardea Photographics* I. R. Beames 12 *BASF* 26 *Maria Bartha* 115 right *Paul Brierley* 177 top *British Telecom* 97,175 top *Burden Neurological Institute, Bristol, U.K.* 75 *Camera Press* 61,168, Les Wilson 84 *Central Office of Information, London* 119,151 *Bruce Coleman Ltd.* Frieder Sauer 76, Paul Wakefield 143 *Colourific* 24 bottom, 217 *Control Data* 155 *Richard Cooke* 188 left *Daily Telegraph Colour Library* Alexander Low 200 *Edinburgh University* 160-61 centre and right *Elizabeth Photo Library* 17, 20, 56, 77, 112 right, 121, 135 top, 173, 188 right *Escher Foundation/SPADEM* 69 bottom *Vivien Fifield* 10 *Ford of Europe* 112 left, 129 top, 185 *Frank Spooner Picture Library* 24 top, 116 *John Frazer, Ulster Polytechnic* 54 *Richard and Sally Greenhill* 7, 27, 43, 156 *Victor Gruen and Associates* 109 *Inmarsat* 175 bottom *International Dias* 216 top *London Scientific Fotos* 147 *Mary Evans Picture Library* 23, 33, 81, 107, 149, 164, *Middlesex Hospital* 146 *Multimedia Publications Inc.* 210, M. Koren 71, 137, 171, 194 right, 203 top, 204 left, 216 bottom left and right *Open University Library* 136 *Pelli, Lumsden, Jacobsen designers* 204 right *Gordon Pask* 78, 92 bottom, 134, 135 bottom left and right, 145, 165 *Rediffusion Simulation Ltd.* 152 *Renault (UK) Ltd.* 114 *Rex Features Ltd.* 33 bottom, 39, 40 top and bottom, 218, Paul Brown 48, Fotos International 41, (George Whitear) 68, (Micklejon) 59, Sipa Press 49 top and bottom, (Frilet) 88 top, (Safa Marry) 88 bottom, (Mingam) 47 *Rockwell International* 28 *Ann Ronan Picture Library* 6, 13 *The Science Museum* 8, 16 *Science Photo Library* 70 *Sinclair* 30 *W. H. Smith* 172 above and below *Rose Spilberg* 47 inset, 122 *Texas Instruments Ltd.* 160 left *John Topham Picture Library* 61, 115 left *University of Pennsylvania* 19 *Vision International* 201 top, Explorer (Duport) 177 bottom, (G. Sommer) 144, Fournier/Explorer (P. H. Anderson) 140, Chris Kapolka 62, Paolo Koch 43, 44, 184, 192, 194 left, 217 bottom right, M. Rosenlund 205, Scala 133, 191 (Henry Moore), Heini Schreebel 22, Anthea Sieveking 87, 153 *John Watney Photo Library* 126 *Komura-Yamaka* 129 *Chris Yates* 196 *Young Artists* Angus Mckie 136, 203 bottom, Stuart Hughes 124 *ZEFA* Big Mike 120, A. Fernandes 169, J. Pfaff 45, G. Sommer 29

Illustrations
Clive Frampton 3-D graphs *Millions Design* artwork and diagrams

Acknowledgements

For permission to quote and excerpt, the authors extend their thanks to:

Margaret Chisman, Creative Computing, Morris Plains, N.J., 1977 (computer verse, page 35)

Computerworld-UK (tables, page 51 and 128)

Time magazine and the American Federation of Information Processing Societies (attitude survey, page 52-53)

Joseph Weizenbaum (ELIZA dialogue, page 90-91)

Terry Winograd (SHRDLU dialogue, page 100-101)

John Evans, The Impact of Microelectronics on Employment in Western Europe in the 1980s, European Trade Union Institute, 1979 (table, page 113)

Ted Nelson, Literary Machines, Ted Nelson, 1981 (diagram, page 123)

A. Payne, B. Hutchings and P. Ayre, Computer Software for Schools, Pitmans, 1980 (VILLAGE dialogue, page 157-158)

T. R. Ide, The Computer and the Communications Revolution, workshop paper for the Club of Rome, February 1981 (graph, page 176)

R. Curnow and S. Curran, The Silicon Factor, National Extension College, UK, 1979 (graph, page 181)

Juan Rada, The Impact of Microelectronics, International Labour Organization, 1980 (bar chart, page 183).